Imaging of Trabecular Microfracture and Bone Marrow Edema and Hemorrhage

Yong-Whee Bahk

Imaging of Trabecular Microfracture and Bone Marrow Edema and Hemorrhage

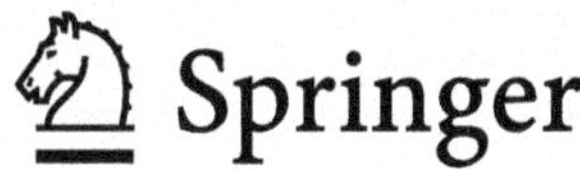

Yong-Whee Bahk
The Catholic University of Korea
School of Medicine Affiliated
Yangji Hospital
Seoul
Korea (Republic of)

ISBN 978-981-15-4465-1 ISBN 978-981-15-4466-8 (eBook)
https://doi.org/10.1007/978-981-15-4466-8

This Springer imprint is published by the registered company Springer Nature Singapore Pte Ltd.
The registered company address is: 152 Beach Road, #21-01/04 Gateway East, Singapore 189721, Singapore

For those who suffer from skeletal diseases and those who heal and help the sufferers

Foreword

Professor Y. W. Bahk, the author of this book, is internationally well recognized as a pioneer in designing and applying advanced bone scintigraphy using pinhole collimation to enhance the sensitivity and specificity of the molecular diagnostic imaging of callused trabecular microfracture to a micrographic level in the whole human body along with the differentiation of bone marrow edema from hemorrhage.

Principally, Prof. Bahk achieved his image micrographic work on the physics of pinhole collimator imaging and biochemistry, for instance, bone metabolism. Metabolic bone change necessarily occurs in osteoneogenesis, and it can be imaged by the tracer-labeled diphosphonates. The results bring off superb diagnostic signal to precisely denote pathology not shown by ordinary imaging modalities. This monograph gives a grand display of the power of his specific imaging technique.

Prof. Bahk initiated his work decades ago by investigating the power of micrographic medical imaging published in the *Journal of Nuclear Medicine* in 1987. It was entitled "Pinhole Collimator Bone Scintigraphy in Differential Diagnosis of Metastasis, Fracture, and Infections of the Spine." It was rightly written to originally highlight the unique nature of pinhole bone scan image which specifically reveals differential pathological changes. The multiple-parallel-hole collimator bone scan cannot demonstrate such a fine detail. Based on the pinhole scan studies, he wrote a book entitled *Combined Scintigraphic and Radiographic Diagnosis of Bone and Joint Diseases* from Springer. The fourth and fifth editions of this book were published that were reinforced by gamma correction interpretation.

Most recently, his decades-long endeavor to develop ^{99m}Tc-HDP pinhole bone scan was upraised by the adoption of gamma correction as referred to in this monograph, and it has become a new stream in bone imaging usefully applied to the micrographic imaging reorientation of ^{99m}Tc-HDP pinhole bone scan. It enabled the demonstration of callused trabecular microfracture (CTMF) with micro-size molecular measurement.

Professor Bahk found that the tiniest CTMF so far demonstrated by gamma correction pinhole bone scan consisted of a single pixel that measures 200 μm in size. He termed this imaging method 99mTc-HDP gamma correction pinhole bone scan (99mHDP GCPBS). Actually, 99mTc-HDP GCPBS can very neatly visualize CTMF, making precise quantification possible in terms of the number of affected pixel(s). A single pixel measures 200 μm in size, and it can be easily measured using a common magnifying optic lens.

By so processing it was confirmed that gamma correction MRI and CT and conventional radiography can efficiently and clearly visualize CTMF. On the other hand, the review of literature revealed that an anatomical study was performed on CTMF in cadavers by Vernon-Roberts and Pirie at the London Hospital in 1973. Their result was used to anatomically validate Prof. Bahk's renovated imaging study on in vivo morpho-biochemical CTMF. The results of all those CTMF studies were so far separately accumulated now needing a corroboratory summation by pictorial presentation along with proposals toward future work as explained in this monograph of micrographic molecular diagnostic imaging.

Ludwig E. Feinendegen
Emeritus Professor of Nuclear Medicine
Heinrich-Heine Düsseldorf University
Düsseldorf, Germany

Preface

Fundamentally, medical diagnostic imaging is based on the anatomy that is systematically enlivened by molecular change, biochemistry, metabolism, and functioning in living human subjects. Hence, the ideal of the medical imaging is to realistically visualize objects with the finest possible anatomical structure which is enriched with in vivo histopathological and physiochemical profiles as finely and neatly as possible. For example, the trabecular microfracture with repair callus formation, the smallest one which measures 200 μm in size or one pixel, would appear to be an ideal object to explore from such a viewpoint. As is well known, the modern clinical medicine and medical science are enriched with plural potent imaging tools including MRI, MDCT, and conventional radiography. Unfortunately, however, the resolution level of all those currently available imaging is in low millimeter range.

The aims of this summarizing monograph of already achieved medical imaging means are primarily to introduce and discuss the basic principle of the ACDSee 10 gamma correction ^{99m}Tc-HDP pinhole bone scan along with the additional attainments through its successful extended application to MRI, conventional radiography, and MDCT. This attempt is hoped to open an avenue to *medical micrometric imaging diagnosis*.

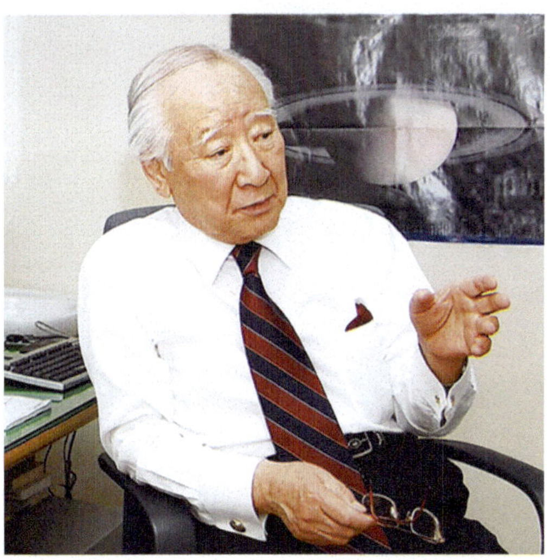

Seoul, Republic of Korea
March 7, 2020

Yong-Whee Bahk

Acknowledgments

I am more than so grateful to Professor Dr. Ludwig Feinendegen for his graceful foreword for my humble book on "Micrographic ACDSee-10 gamma correction medical imaging." I also would like to acknowledge Dr. Chul-Soo Kim, M.D., Ph.D., the Chairman of Yangji Hospital, Seoul, for his kind concern on and support for this study during the past 3 years.

Many thanks are due to Mr. Woo-Jin Chang, the librarian of the Catholic University Uijeongbu St. Mary's Hospital for his expertise bibliographic work, Mr.Younghwan Kim of Korea Siemens healthnier Company for his updated medical imaging technology information, and Ms. Lauren Kim of Seoul Springer-Nature for her sincere and devoted services.

Finally, I would like to pay a special and hearty tribute to my wife Rosa Yeun-Soo, sons and daughter, and their spouses and seven grandchildren for everything we have always shared hand-in-hand during all these prolong perspiring, endeavoring, and inspiring years.

Contents

Contributors

Jeongmi Park, MD, PhD Department of Radiology, Yoido St. Mary's Hospital, The Korea Catholic University Medical School, Seoul, Korea

Jeasoo Kim, PhD Department of Ocean Engineering, Korea Maritime and Ocean University, Busan, Korea

Yong An Chung, MD, PhD Department of Nuclear Medicine and Radiology, Inchon St. Mary's Hospital, The Korea Catholic University Medical School, Inchon, Korea

Jiwon Bahk, BSc Department of Physics, Sejong University, Seoul, Korea

Introduction

1

As well-known medical imaging science was naturally born in the moment of the discovery of X-ray by W. C. Röntgen in November of 1895 in Würzburg and decades afterward it was followed by the clinical nuclear medicine initiated by H. L. Blumgart of the Thorndike Memorial Laboratory of the Boston City Hospital and Harvard University who measured pulmonary circulation time using radium (Blumgart and Weiss 1928). Unnoticedly thereafter, 45 years elapsed before the epoch-making computed tomography (CT) was invented by G. N. Hounsfield of England in 1972. The discovery was enabled by the construction of a huge computer. Successively, magnetic resonance imaging (MRI) was constructed by P. Mansfield in 1975. Thence, these triumphant medical imaging techniques became to overwhelm and they once appeared to hush conventional radiography (CR) and basic ^{99m}Tc-HDP pinhole bone scanning of bone and joint. Recently, however, with the good use of gamma correction, the upgraded ACDSee 10 in particular, the current trend in medical bone imaging appears to have advantageously moved toward the revival of not only conventional radiography but also ^{99m}Tc-HDP pinhole bone scan due to up-to-dated *micrographic imaging* that enabled the demonstration of callused trabecular microfracture (CTMF) and even its quantitation. Advantageously, the author noted that the smallest CTMF so imaged to consist of single pixel, which measures as small as 200 μm in size. This imaging was termed ^{99m}Tc-HDP gamma correction pinhole bone scan (^{99m}Tc-HDP GCPBS) (Fig. 1.1) (Bahk et al. 2010). ^{99m}Tc-HDP GCPBS neatly shows CTMF making precise quantitation possible in terms of pixel. A single pixel was 200 μm in size, which could be measured mathematically (Jung et al. 2016) or using a magnifying lens. Thus, it was proven to be more than necessary now to import the gamma correction to MRI and CT and conventional radiography to diagnostically reinforce MRI and CT and to revitalize CR to precisely diagnose CTMF.

Review of literature disclosed a basic anatomical study, which was performed on the callused trabecular microfractures (CTMF) of the lumbar vertebrae in the post mortem subjects at the London Hospital in 1973 by Vernon-Roberts and Pirie (Fig. 1.2a). In the latest refined imaging study on the in vivo morpho-biochemical CTMF, the beneficial use of their pioneering in vitro anatomic work was made as a useful anatomical validation source of ^{99m}Tc-HDP GCPBS study (Fig. 1.2b). Actually, their in vitro study played an important verification role for the imaging of CTMF, which is characterized by unsuppressed high ^{99m}Tc-HDP uptake (Bahk et al. 2010). Preliminarily, we performed an experimental histological study on endosteal rimming inflicted in the femoral shaft of young rats by the naturally falling iron-ball contusion method (Fig. 1.3) (Gläser et al. 2011). The results of all those studies on CTMF were so far accumulated rather

Y.-W. Bahk, *Imaging of Trabecular Microfracture and Bone Marrow Edema and Hemorrhage*,
https://doi.org/10.1007/978-981-15-4466-8_1

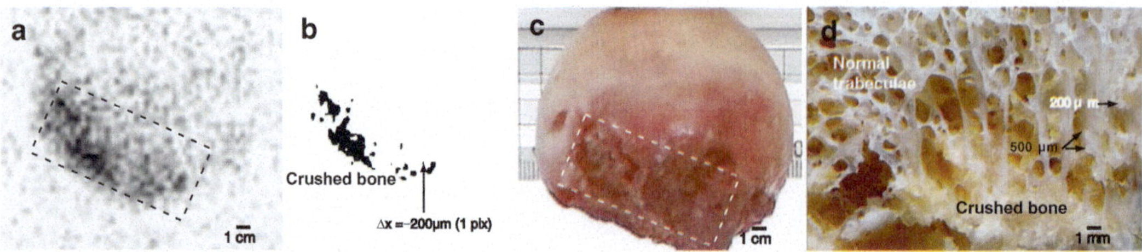

Fig. 1.1 ACDSee-10 gamma correction pinhole bone scan demonstration and quantification of callused trabecular microfractures (CTMF). (**a**) Naïve ^{99m}Tc-HDP pinhole scan shows nonspecific blurry tracer uptake (*frame*). (**b**) Gamma correction pinhole bone scan can highlight single pixel CTMF measuring 200 μm in size. (**c**) Surgical specimen shows microfractures in femoral neck fracture (*frame*). (**d**) Surface microscopy of neck fracture shows CTMF along with crushed bone and normal trabeculae

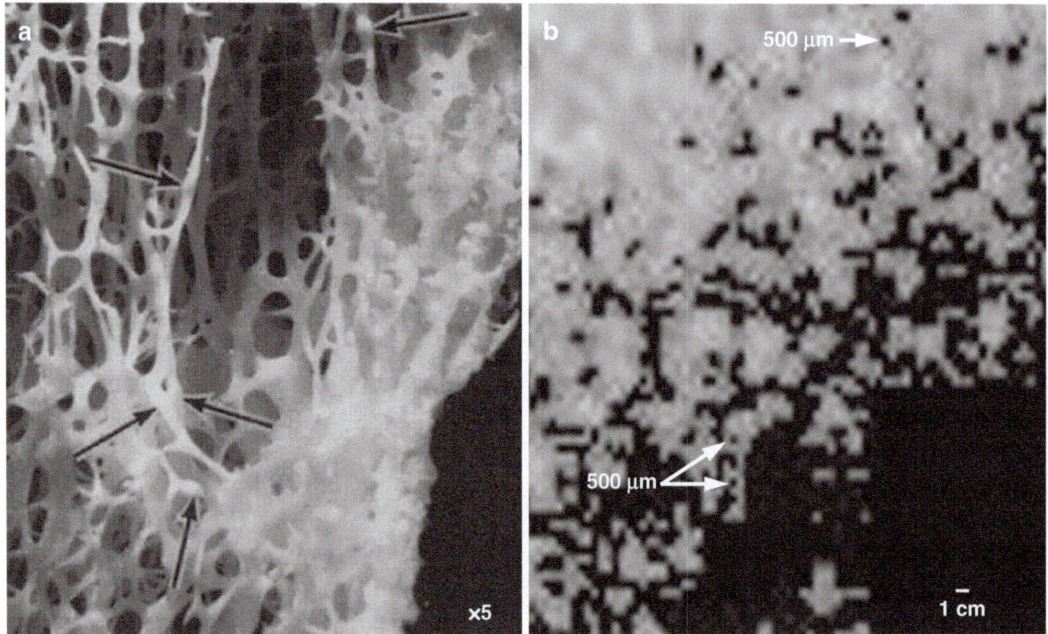

Fig. 1.2 Unique in vitro anatomical and in vivo ^{99m}Tc-HDP bone scintigraphic demonstrations of trabecular microfractures in vertebral body. (**a**) Vernom-Roberts and Pirie of London Hospital published in 1973 microfractures in macerated L4 vertebral body (with permission). It measured up to 0.5 mm in size. (**b**) Recently, we were able to image microcalluses using ACDSee-7 gamma correction ^{99m}Tc-HDP pinhole scan (arrows). It is an in vivo *micrographic* imaging means to specifically and demonstrate trabecular microfractures with biochemical information on osteoneogenesis. It is with penumbra measuring 0.5 mm in size

independently now needing corroboratory summarization through pictorial case presentation, discussion, conclusion, and futuristic proposition in this monographic book of *micrographic medical imaging*.

The aims of this monograph are to describe and openly discuss the theories, methods, and practical clinical diagnostic usefulness of gamma correction imaging in the form of (1) gamma correction ^{99m}Tc-HDP pinhole bone scan, (2) gamma correction MRI, (3) gamma correction CT, and (4) even gamma correction conventional radiography. It is a refreshing interest that the almost neglected and nearly forgotten radiography can

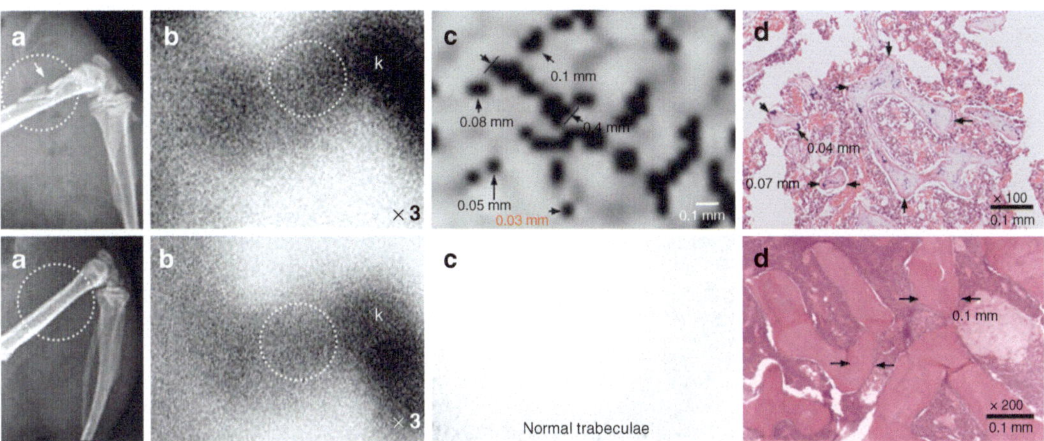

Fig. 1.3 Experimental endosteal rimming incited by falling iron-ball hemorrhagic contusion and normal control in young rats. Top panel: (**a**) falling iron-ball induced fracture is seen (circle). (**b**) Threefold magnified pinhole scan shows trauma hypocenter (circle). (**c**) Gamma correction PBS shows unsuppressed tracer uptake in trabecular endosteal rimming. (**d**) H&E stain (×100) shows endosteal rimming and diffuse hemorrhage (arrows). Bottom panel: (**a**) normal control radiograph. (**b**) Threefold magnified pinhole scan shows the control area (circle). (**c**) Gamma correction pinhole bone scan shows clean suppression of tracer uptake. (**d**) H&E stain (×100) is negative

now be made anew revived as a highly refined, useful, informative imaging tool of the fine anatomical demonstration and precise, convenient quantitation of CTMF in the form of gamma correction ^{99m}Tc-HDP pinhole bone scanning and MRI. Actually, we realized that, unlike ACDSee-7, ACDSee-10 gamma correction radiography can very finely depict CTMF like ^{99m}Tc-HDP pinhole bone scan does but not providing bone metabolic information in terms of ^{99m}Tc-HDP uptake. The radiographic demonstration of callused microtrabecular change is well comparable to that of CT although the former is a 3D image and the latter is a 2D image. It is to be mentioned here in passing that microfocus-CT can microscopically visualize bone trabeculae, but it is clinically only limitedly used in an in vitro study (Hutchinson et al. 2017). As a matter of fact, MRI is currently used widely for the fine demonstration of not only bone and joint but also a number of intra- and periarticular juxtaosseous soft tissue structures such as ligament, tendon, synovium, and muscle. Regrettably, however, it is yet unable for MRI to provide the precise metabolic profile of the osteoneogenesis in acute CTMF. In regard to the precision level the size of the smallest CTMF imaged by ACDSee-10 gamma correction is 200 μm (unit pixel) (Fig. 1.4). It is considered that this is a primitive initiation of an in vivo medical imaging of injured bone trabeculae like primitive light microscope.

Gamma correction ^{99m}Tc-HDP pinhole bone scan can now distinguish blurry edema and hemorrhage with meager ^{99m}Tc-HDP uptake (Fig. 1.5a) from the trabecular fracture with strong tracer uptake which is characteristically unsuppressed by gamma correction (Fig. 1.5b), but the contrast medium used in MRI may obscure important anatomical detail preventing the fine diagnosis of microfracture (Fig. 1.5d). Nevertheless, however, when MRI is judiciously processed using gamma correction CTMF can be successfully imaged finely (Fig. 1.6). Practically, gamma correction MRI can neatly highlight and demonstrate CTMF without penumbra when ACDSee-10 version is used (Fig. 1.7c). We found that the gamma correction is easy to perform and is highly economical. Actually, the smallest callused microfracture measures 200 μm in size. Very importantly, it is here to be remarked that the micrometric size of CTMF in this study derived from the basic scale of < – > which measures 1 mm in length consisting of 5 pixels in the x-axis on the computer screen. Thus, one pixel on this scale measures 200 μm in size.

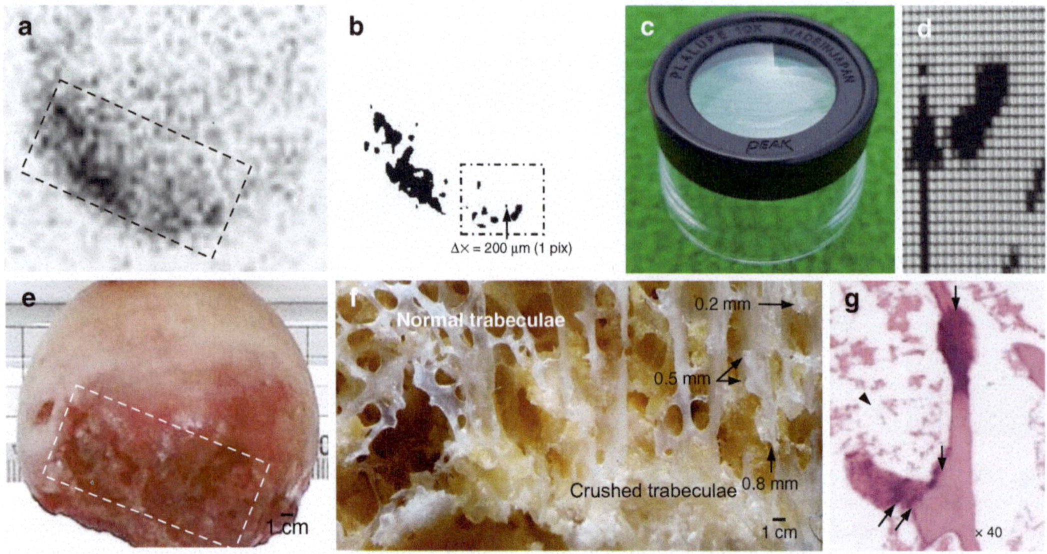

Fig. 1.4 ACDSee-10 gamma correction ^{99m}Tc-HDP pinhole bone scan demonstration and magnifying lens measurement of 200-µm callused trabecular microfracture. Microfracture is imaged with dark microspotty tracer uptake on gamma correction pinhole bone scan. (**a**) Naïve pinhole scan shows nonspecific blurry ^{99m}Tc-HDP uptake in microfractures (frame). (**b**) Gamma correction pinhole scan shows multiple trabecular microfractures with the smallest measuring 200 µm in size. Δ*x* is *x*-axis. (**c**) 10× magnifying lens. (**d**) Hand phone camera snap shows single pixel involvement. (**e**) Fresh surgical specimen shows microfractures in the femoral neck (frame). (**f**) Surgical surface microscopic view of framed portion shows typical seed-pearly calluses. (**h**) H&E stain shows a characteristic base stain in microfractures in a trabeculae

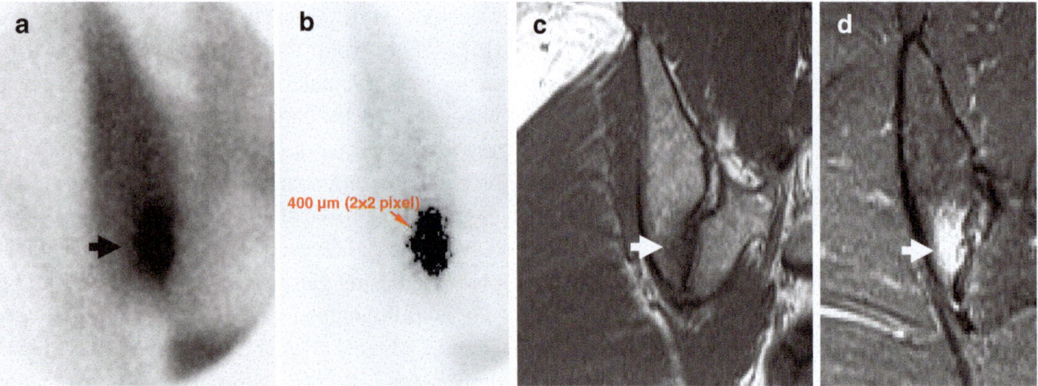

Fig. 1.5 Sacrotuberous ligament enthesitis with fractures in a 29-year-old male badminton player who had acute painful strain in the right lower sacroiliac joint. MRI cannot distinguish fracture from tendinitis. (**a**) Posterior pinhole scan shows a blurry ovoid area of intense ^{99m}Tc-HDP uptake in the lower aspect of the sacroiliac joint (*arrow*). (**b**) ACDSee-10 gamma correction view shows the suppression of blurry tracer uptake highlighting intense tracer uptake in trabecular fractures. There is a callused microfracture measuring 400 µm (2×2 pixels) in size. (**c, d**) T1-weightged (500/10) and contrast enhanced T1-weighted (772/9) MR images show low signal intensity and positive contrast enhancement at the insertion of upper fibers of sacrotuberous ligament, respectively. No fractures shown due to contrast enhancement (*arrow*)

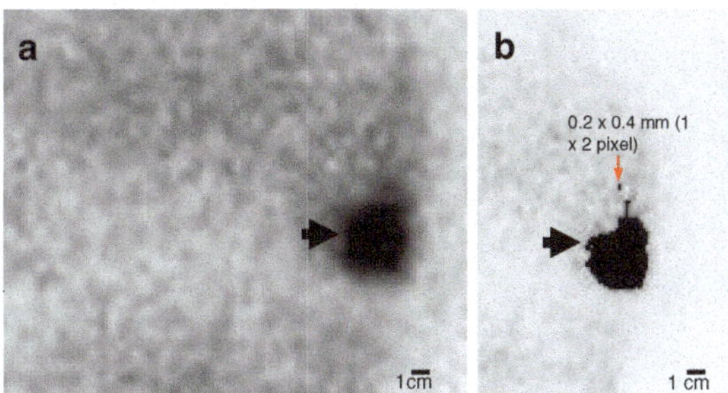

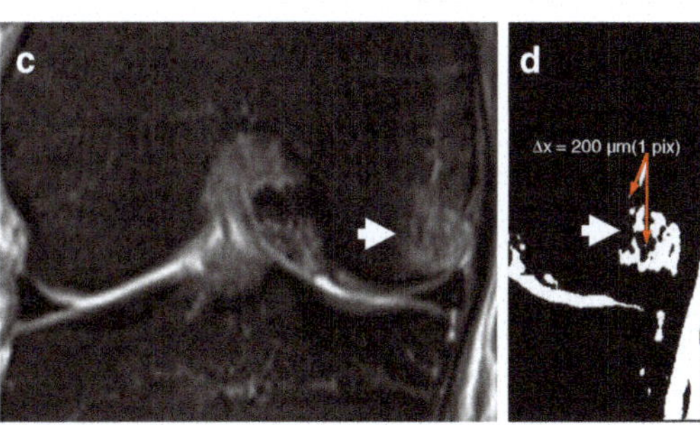

Fig. 1.6 ACDSee-10 enhanced gamma correction ^{99m}Tc-HDP pinhole scan shows a round traumatic injury in the right medial femoral condyle incited by motor vehicle accident in a 55-year-old male. (**a**) Naïve ^{99m}Tc-HDP pinhole scan shows blurry round tracer uptake (*arrow*). (**b**) Enhanced gamma correction pinhole scan shows sharply defined geographic fracture (*large arrow*) with a dash-shaped and 200 × 450 μm microfractures (*small arrow*). (**c**) Naïve coronal T2 WT FS MR image (3,500/18) shows a 1-cm lesion (*arrow*). (**d**) Gamma correction MR image shows injury to consist of multiple sharply defined speckled fractures including two 200-μm microcalluses (*arrows*)

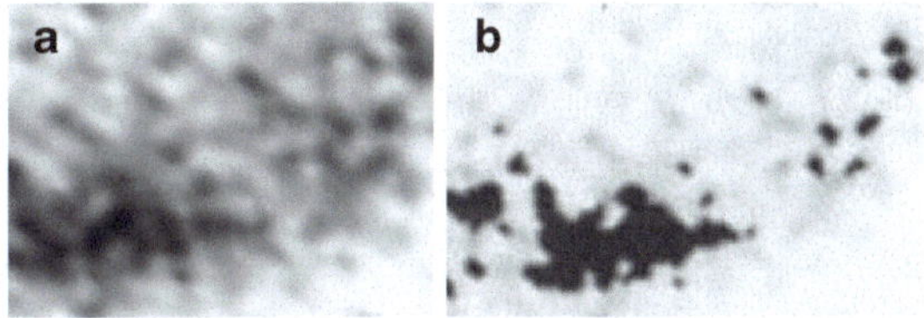

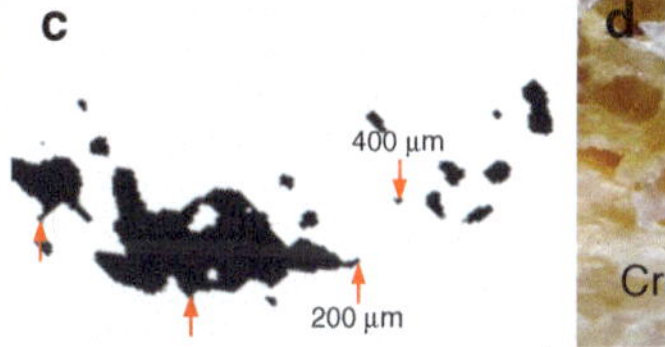

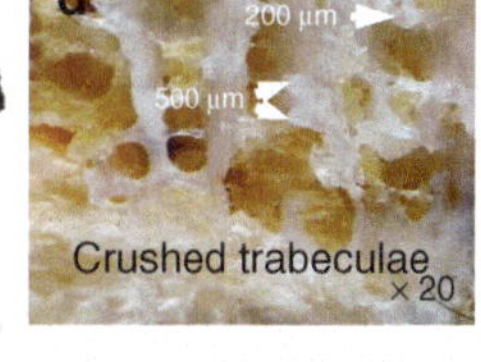

Fig. 1.7 Neat definition and higher sensitivity of ACDSee-10 gamma correction image compared to conventional ACDSee-7 gamma correction with histological validation in surgically removed femoral head for bipolar prosthesis in a 72-year-old female patient. (**a**) Naïve ^{99m}Tc-HDP pinhole scan shows nonspecific blurry tracer uptake. (**b**) ACDSee-7 gamma correction pinhole scan shows micro and archipelagic fractures with penumbra. (**c**) ACDSee-10 gamma correction view shows neatly sharpened microfracture contour (red arrows). Smaller calluses are additively demonstrated because of increased image sensitivity. The smallest one measures 200 μm (single pixel) in size. (**d**) Surface microscope of ROI shows seed-pearly trabecular microfractures and a 200μm microfracture and large crushed trabeculae

CT and MRI, incepted in the early 1970s, have promisingly burgeoned under the influence of then uniquely developed conventional radiography which could already securely visualize microtrabeculae (Fig. 1.8) although early primitive CT was unable to do so (Fig. 1.9a). In the meantime, both modalities have rapidly achieved technological development so that their latest models can successfully demonstrate refined microtrabeculae (Fig. 1.9b). Figure 1.10 assuredly demonstrates the finely depicted trabeculae in a conventional radiograph, CT, and MRI. Unfortunately, however, such a breakthrough was a partial success as it was not sufficient to convincingly visualize CTMF (callused trabecular microfracture). Hence, we sought imaging means to specifically visualize injured trabeculae eventually finding *gamma correction*, which can neatly highlight and specifically diagnose CTMF. Naturally, we made an attempt to import gamma correction not only to ^{99m}Tc-HDP pinhole bone scan but also to MRI, CT, and conventional radiograph to specifically image CTMF. Technically, the gamma correction was extended as a "wizard" tool to most clinical diagnostic imaging modalities and at last, we have become to finely visualize CTMF and to additionally differentiate bone marrow edema and hemorrhage and trabecular microfracture (Fig. 1.11) (Bahk et al. 2019). GCPBS proved that mild physiological bone tracer uptake, the source of disturbing image blur or penumbra in normal and damaged trabeculae, can be efficiently eliminated simply using gamma

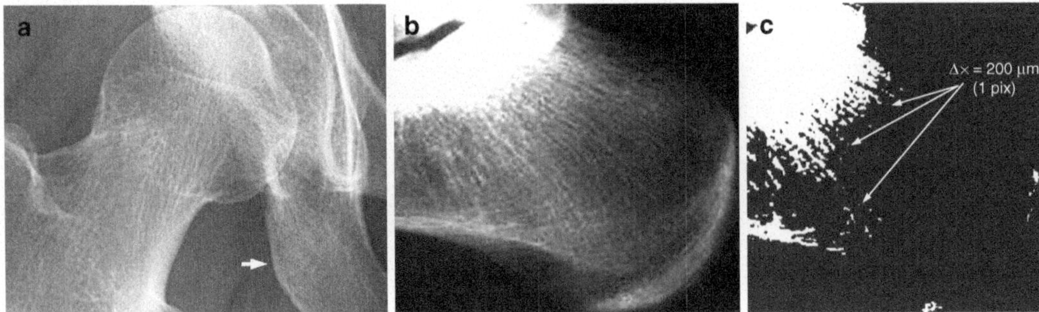

Fig. 1.8 Demonstration of well-developed normal trabeculae in the bones of the main weight-bearing femoral head and neck in the hip and calcaneus in the heel in adults. Trabeculae are typically arranged along the lines of major stress and strain. (**a**) Anteroposterior radiograph of the right hip shows well-developed trabeculae in the femoral head and neck but not in the ischium which is out of major stress line (arrow). (**b**) Mediolateral radiograph of the right hindfoot demonstrates well-developed obliquely arranged trabeculae. (**c**) ACDSee-10 gamma correction radiograph shows trabecular microcalluses with the smallest one measuring 200 μm in size

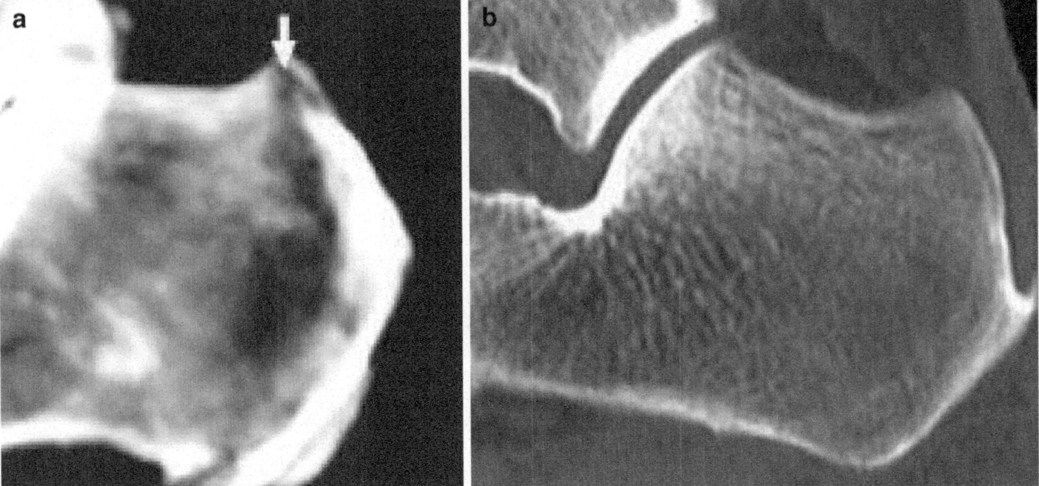

Fig. 1.9 Rapid improvement of image quality of CT over a period of one decade. (**a**) Early CT could hardly image trabeculae demonstrating barely discernible rough unresolved trabeculae and a large fracture (arrow). (**b**) In the meantime, CT achieved rapid technological development and image refinement so that the late model became to successfully visualize trabeculae

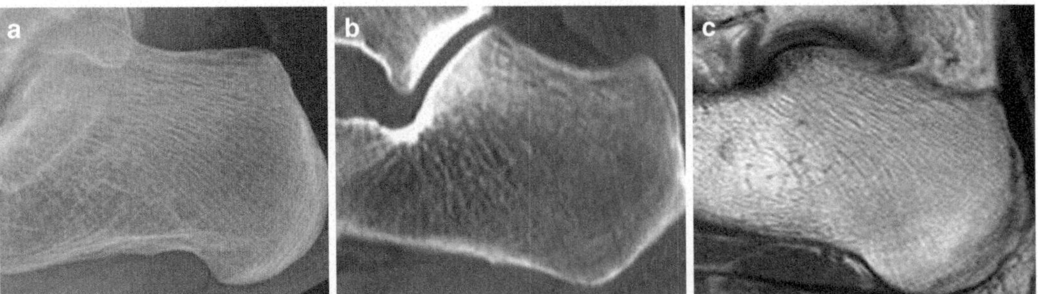

Fig. 1.10 Difference in image resolution of conventional radiograph, MDCT, and 1.5T MRI. (**a**) Radiograph shows the most fine bright thready trabeculae. (**b**) CT shows less fine bright trabeculae. (**c**) MRI demonstrates fine dark trabeculae. Subjects are all in the third decade

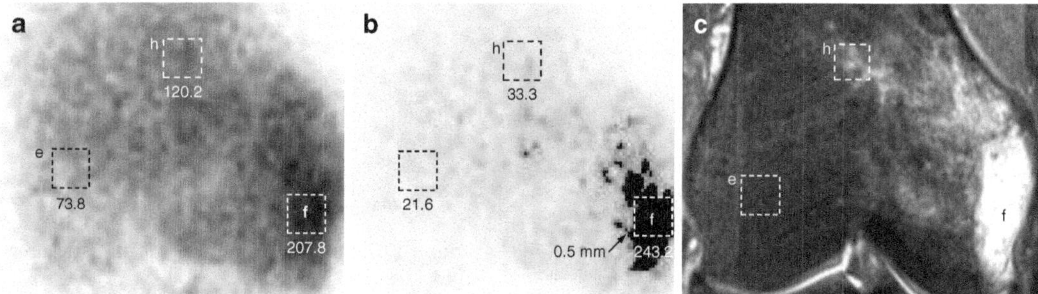

Fig. 1.11 Edema and hemorrhage can be differentiated using ACDSee-7 GCPBS and NIH ImageJ densitometry. This is a simplified view to specifically feature the suppressed tracer uptake in edema and hemorrhage and highlighted ^{99m}Tc-HDP uptake in fractures. (**a**) Naïve pinhole scan shows three 1-cm^2 areas of blurry tracer uptake of edema (*e*) and hemorrhage (*h*), and fracture (*f*) with AU value, which was 73.8 in edema, 120.2 in hemorrhage, 207 in fracture. (**b**) The gamma correction did suppress edema and hemorrhage uptake highlighting fractures (*f*). The smallest fracture measured 0.5 mm. (**c**) Corroborative FS coronal T2-weighted MR image (3500/18) shows a 1-cm^2 area of hemorrhage (*h*) with bright signal intensity and another 1-cm^2 area of edema with barely discernible bright signal intensity (*e*)

correction. It is to be noted that trabeculae are imaged as a fine bright linear structure on CT and radiograph, but contrary as fine dark linear structures in MR image (Fig. 1.10c).

This monograph is aimed at systematic and holistic presentation, discussion, and summarization of what have been observed and achieved from so far performed clinical studies and one rat experimentation on gamma correction ^{99m}Tc-HDP pinhole bone scan, MRI, CR, and CT of normal and pathological bone trabeculae in series (Bahk et al. 2016). As mentioned, Vernon-Roberts and Pirie anatomically explored trabecula and microcallus in cadaveric lumbar specimens in 1973 (Vernon-Roberts and Pirie 1973) (Fig. 1.2). According to them CTMF measured up to 0.5 mm in thickness. It implies that a trabecula per se without callus measures less than 0.5 mm in adult, presumably denoting that un-callused trabeculae measures from 200 to 300 μm in thickness. Characteristically, the meager ^{99m}Tc-HDP uptake in intact trabecula is suppressed by gamma correction (Fig. 1.12c), but contrarily and impressively the tracer uptake in actively forming CTMF is unsuppressed because of active osteoneogenesis (Fig. 1.12f). The similar phenomenon is confirmed to occur in MRI (Fig. 1.13), CT (Fig. 1.14), and conventional radiograph (Fig. 1.15). The suppression of the tracer uptake in trabeculae on GCPBS is a confirmative evidence of that there is no fracture with osteoneogenesis. The unsuppressed ^{99m}Tc-HDP uptake in microfracture is due to the avid chemical incorporation of ^{99m}Tc-HDP into amorphous calcium phosphate in injured bone, whereas the suppressed bone tracer uptake in edema and hemorrhage is due to tracer adhesion to crystalline hydroxyapatite (Francis et al. 1980). It is to be noted that GCPBS is useful not only to qualitatively highlight a trabecular image but also to quantitatively measure the size of callused trabecular fractures. The size can be measured either mathematically using pixelized measurement method (Jung et al. 2016) or simply by the direct counting of involved pixel using a magnifying optic lens (Fig. 1.4). Actually, the smallest CTMF measured by pixel calculation method was 230 μm and measured by the magnifying lens counting method was 200 μm.

The term trabecula derived from Latin *trabs* which means beam. Anatomically, trabeculae not only support the bone integrity but also provide labyrinthine space to richly house blood-forming marrow tissues and others. Recently, gamma correction has become usefully imported to pinhole bone scanning (Fig. 1.11) (Bahk et al. 2019) and extendedly also to MRI (Fig. 1.13), CT (Fig. 1.14), and conventional radiograph (Fig. 1.15) all highly

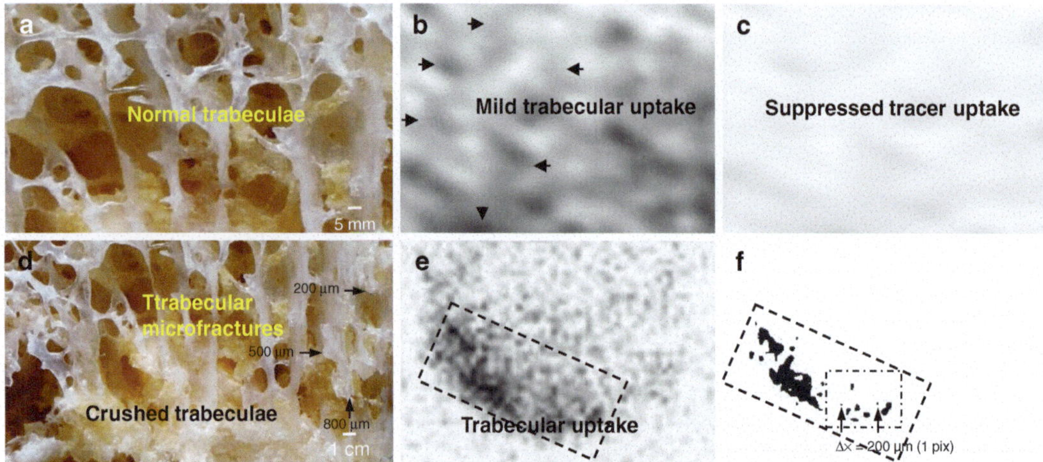

Fig. 1.12 NIH ImageJ densitometry intensity value of ^{99m}Tc-HDP uptake in histopathologically verified normal trabeculae in surgically removed femoral head for bipolar prosthesis in a 72-year-old female patient. (**a**) Twofold magnified surgical micrograph shows normal trabeculae (arrows). (**b**) Naïve pinhole bone scan of normal trabeculae shows blurry nonspecific tracer uptake, which was calculated as ≤50 AU (arrows) (Bahk et al. 2019). (**c**) Gamma correction suppresses tracer uptake in normal trabeculae. (**d**) Surgical micrograph of shows callused trabecular microfractures (arrows). (**e**) Naïve pinhole scan shows nonspecific blurry tracer uptake. (**f**) Gamma correction view shows two archipelagic fractures and multiple microfractures with the smallest one measuring 200 μm in size

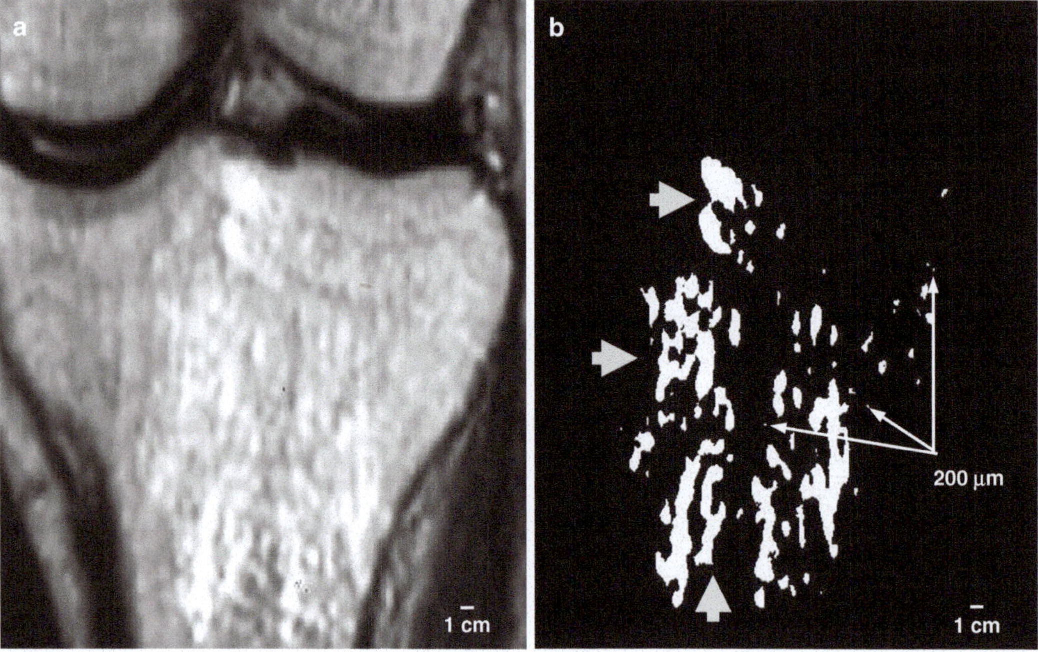

Fig. 1.13 Remarkable callused trabecular microfractures in the right tibial tuberosity incited by bicycle accident in a 78-year-old male. (**a**) Naïve T2 weighted (3500/85) FS coronal MR image shows extensive nonspecific blurry bright signal intensities. (**b**) In contrast, however, ACDSee-10 gamma correction can neatly highlight archipelagic and mottled callused microcalluses (short arrows). In addition, the gamma correction can sensitively visualize 200-μm microcalluses (long arrows)

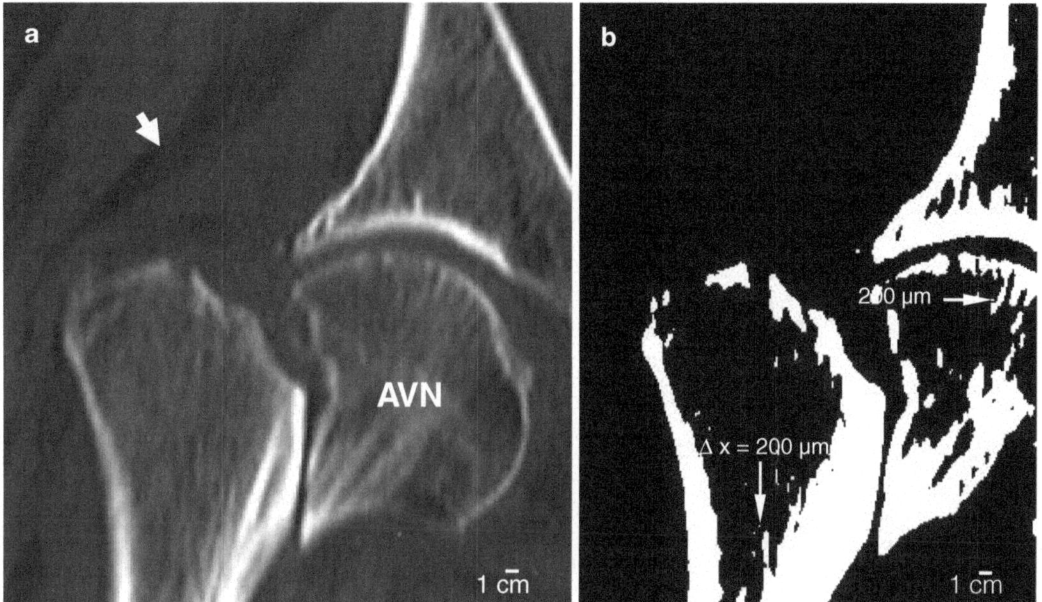

Fig. 1.14 Vertically fissuring right femoral neck fracture with avascular necrosis of the femoral head (AVN) due to falling down from sleeping bed in a 92-year-old male. (**a**) Naïve CT shows gaping femoral neck fracture along with joint capsule distension (*arrow*). (**b**) ACDSee-10 gamma correction view demonstrates multiple callused trabecular microfractures with the smallest ones measuring 200 μm in size (*arrow*)

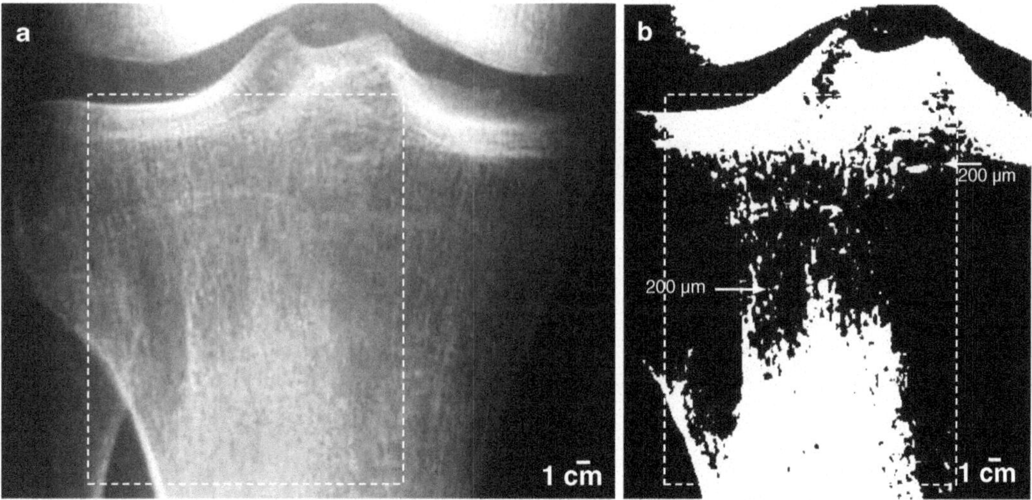

Fig. 1.15 Fine ACDSee-10 gamma correction radiographic demonstration of callused trabecular microfractures in the right proximal tibial metadiaphysis due to motor vehicle contusion in a 57-year-old male. (**a**) Naïve radiograph shows thinning and aggregation of trabeculae (*frame*). (**b**) Gamma correction radiograph shows condensed trabeculae with numerous seed-pearly callused trabecular microfractures (*frame*). The smallest ones measure 200 μm in size (*arrows*)

raising in-vivo medical imaging diagnostic level. The results of such studies are detailed in the following Case Presentation of Chap. 5.

References

Bahk YW, Jeon HS, Kim JM, et al. A novel use of gamma correction for precise ^{99m}Tc-HDP pinhole bone scan diagnosis and classification of knee occult fractures. Skeletal Radiol. 2010;39:807–81.

Bahk YW, Chung YA, Lee UY, et al. Gamma correction ^{99m}Tc-hydroxymethylene diphosphonate pinhole bone scan diagnosis and histopathological verification of trabecular contusion in young rat. Nucl Med communications 2016;37:988–91.

Bahk YW, Kim EE, Chung YA, et al. Precise differential diagnosis of acute bone marrow edema and hemorrhage and trabecular microfractures using naïve and gamma correction pinhole bone scans. J Int Med Res. 2019; https://doi.org/10.1177/0300060518819910.

Blumgart HL, Weiss S. Clinical studies on the velocity of blood flow: IX. The pulmonary circulation time, the velocity of venous blood flow to the heart, and related aspects of the circulation in patient with cardiovascular disease. J Clin Invest. 1928;5:343–77.

Francis MD, Ferguson DL, Tofe AJ, et al. Comparative evaluation of three diphosphonates: in vitro adsorption (C-14 labeled) and in vivo osteogenic uptake (Tc-99m complexed). J Nucl Med. 1980;21:1185–9.

Gläser N, Kneubuehl BP, Zuber S, et al. Biomechanical examination of blunt trauma due to baseball bat blows to the head. J Forensic Biomech. 2011;b2:F100601.

Hutchinson JC, Shelmerdine S, Simcock I, et al. Early clinical applications for imaging at microscopic detail: microfocus computed tomography (micro-CT). Br J Radiol. 2017;90:0113.

Jung JT, Cheon GJ, Lee YS, et al. Pixelized measurement of ^{99m}Tc-HDP micro particles formed in gamma correction phantom pinhole scan: a reference study. Nucl Med Mol Imaging. 2016;50:207–12.

Röntgen WC. On a new kind of radiation (Ueber eine neue Art von Strahlen). Proceedings of Physics-Medical Society of Würzburg 1895; 10.

Vernon-Roberts B, Pirie CJ. Healing trabecular microfractures in the bodies of lumbar vertebrae. Ann Rheum Dis. 1973;32:406–12.

^{99m}Tc-HDP Pinhole Bone Scanning 2

^{99m}Tc-HDP (hydroxymethylene diphosphonate) pinhole bone scanning is an ordinary bone imaging technique upgraded by the additional use of a 4-mm aperture pinhole collimator (Bahk et al. 1987; Kim et al. 1999). However, its remarkably enriched image contents are clinically well demonstrated and histopathologically proven beyond question. Indeed, one may at once recognize that the image contents of pinhole scan are "too different" from those of the parallel hole collimator scan when tested by gamma correction (Fig. 2.1) (Bahk et al. 1987). Indeed, there is a radical difference between the findings of parallel-hole and pinhole collimator scans. For example, in vertebral compression fracture parallel-hole scan shows just a block-like ^{99m}Tc-HDP uptake, but pinhole scan shows intense tracer uptake sharply localized to the L3 upper endplate, which is slightly compressed. The parallel-hole bone scan of infective spondylitis also shows the same block-like tracer uptake in L3 vertebra, but again pinhole scan shows the entirely different finding of apposing tracer uptake in the L2 lower and L3 upper endplates. This is a case of acute infective spondylitis. Essentially, such a difference is resulted from the shaper and finer imaging feasibility of pinhole collimator. It is not related at all with the simple image size enlargement. Very importantly, it is further to be realized that the gamma correction does not work in the parallel bone scan as in pinhole scan (Fig. 2.2). Gamma correction is practically useless in multiple parallel-hole ^{99m}Tc-HDP bone scan.

Basically, ^{99m}Tc-HDP bone scanning is attained by the cumulative consequence of multiple physical and chemical factors including radiopharmaceutical, radioactivity, collimator, detector, and image display and recording devices Technically, ancillary factors such as patient movement during scanning and various technical artifacts can unfavorably affect image qualities in terms of contrast and sensitivity more often than not seriously hindering pathology detection ultimately leading to occasional incorrect diagnosis. The radiotracer must selectively accumulate in bone trabeculae delivering a low possible radiation dose while permitting high count density. In this connection, the half-life of 6.02 h and the monoenergetic 140-keV gamma ray emission of ^{99m}Technetium (^{99m}Tc) labeled to phosphates is an ideal agent for bone scanning. Intravenously injected 740–925 MBq (20–25 mCi) of ^{99m}Tc-HDP in ordinary adult and slightly higher doses in the elderly subject with reduced bone metabolism is considered appropriate.

Y.-W. Bahk, *Imaging of Trabecular Microfracture and Bone Marrow Edema and Hemorrhage*,
https://doi.org/10.1007/978-981-15-4466-8_2

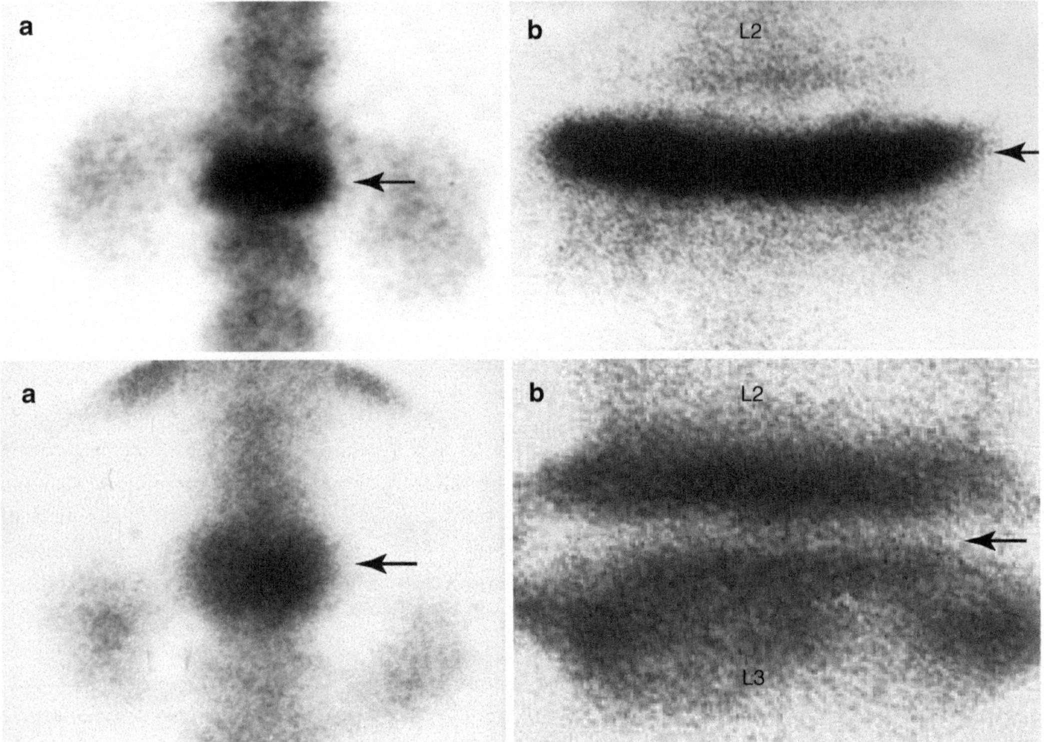

Fig. 2.1 Radical difference between findings of parallel-hole and pinhole collimator scintigraphs. Top panel: (**a**) Parallel-hole scan shows just block-like ^{99m}Tc-HDP uptake in L3 vertebra. (**b**) Pinhole scan, however, shows intense tracer uptakes sharply localized to the L3 upper endplate with mild compression. This is a compression fracture. Bottom panel: (**a**) Parallel-hole scan again shows block-like uptake in L3 vertebra which is just the same as the finding shown in the top panel case. (**b**) Pinhole scan, however, shows an entirely different finding of apposing tracer uptake in the L2 lower and L3 upper endplates. This is acute pyogenic spondylitis. Such an obvious difference is essentially considered to be related to the shaper and finer imaging feasibility of pinhole collimators. It is not related at all with the simple image size enlargement

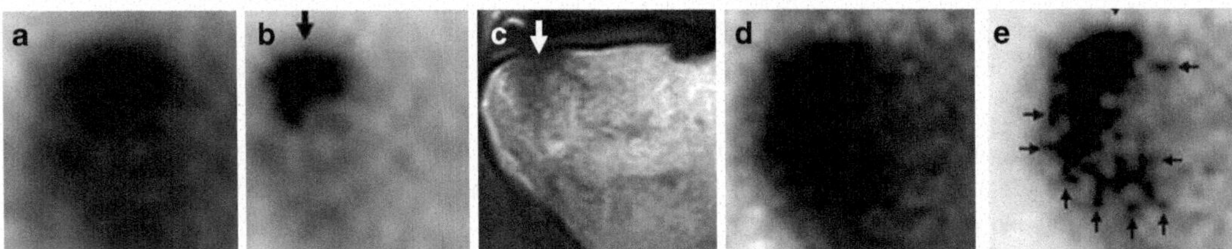

Fig. 2.2 Basically different arboriform fracture presentations in gamma correction multiparallel-hole scan and gamma correction pinhole scan. (**a, b**) Pre- and post-gamma correction parallel hole scans of branching fracture in the lateral tibial condyle of the right tibia shows geographic lesion without any branching at all. (**c**) T1-weighted (460/26) MR image shows a typical branching fracture (arrow). (**d**) Naïve pinhole scan shows non-specific homogeneous tracer uptake (arrow). (**e**) Amazingly, however, the gamma correction view shows an arboriform fracture. The fracture demonstration is far more distinct on 3D pinhole scan than on 2D MR image

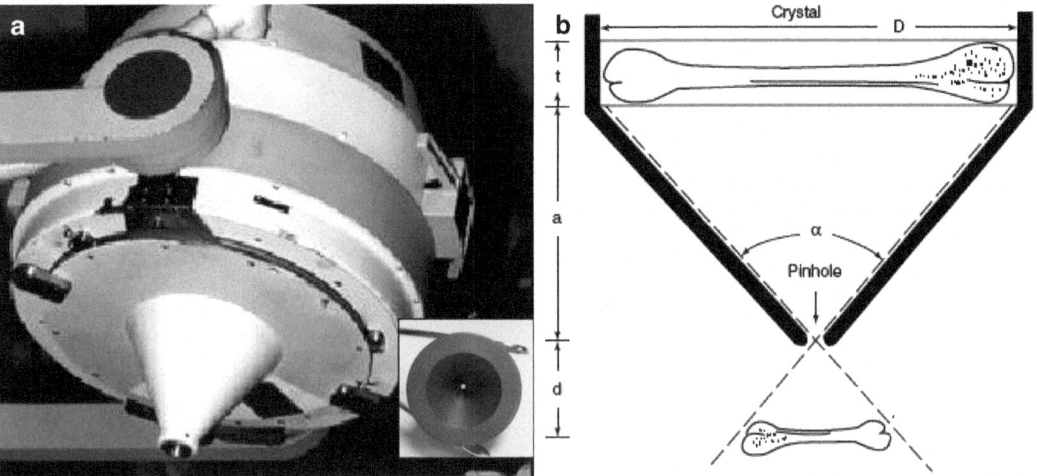

Fig. 2.3 A gamma camera head. (**a**) Compact gamma detector with a pinhole collimator. Inset is a 2-mm pinhole collimator made of tungsten. (**b**) Diagram of the interior structure shows inversion and magnification of pinhole image. **D** Diameter of detector crystal, **t** thickness of detector, **a** collimator height, **d** aperture-to-object distance, and **α** acceptance angle

Technically, a gamma camera system consists of a scintillation detector with collimator, electronic devices, and recording tools. Of these, the size of collimator hole is the most important single variable which directly affects scan image resolution or image quality. Pinhole collimator directs the gamma rays emitted from a selected source in objective to scintillation detector in a specifically designed manner (Fig. 2.3). Actually, four different types of collimators are clinically available: they are pinhole and parallel, converging, and diverging multihole collimators. The pinhole collimator is a cone-shaped heavy metal shield that tapers into a small aperture perforated at the tip which is circular in shape. As shown in Fig. 2.3b pinhole magnification is the actual geometric enlargement of image size and contents like lens magnification or light microscope.

Pinhole aperture size varies from 1 to 8 mm. The aperture size of the pinhole collimator is the topmost important determinant of scan resolution and sensitivity. Understandably, the smaller aperture pinhole collimator produces a scanned image with higher resolution at the expense of sensitivity and vice versa. Accordingly, the optimization of the two contradicting parameters was necessary. In clinical practice, we found that a collimator with an aperture diameter of 4 mm is optimal. The magnification, resolution, and sensitivity of the pinhole scan image may also vary due to the aperture-to-target distance. The image magnification with true gain in resolution can be attained by approximating the collimator tip to the target as close as possible. Basically, the suitability of pinhole scan largely depends on the size of the target to be imaged. We found anatomical structures or organs not larger than 10 cm in size are good objects to examine using pinhole scanning. Such objects are actually all axial and appendicular bones in adults. Indeed, a portion or the whole of large structures such as the skull, spine, chest, long bones, and pelvis can be snugly imaged attaining markedly enriched diagnostic information (Figs. 2.4, 2.5, and 2.6). When processed by *gamma correction*, pinhole bone scan becomes

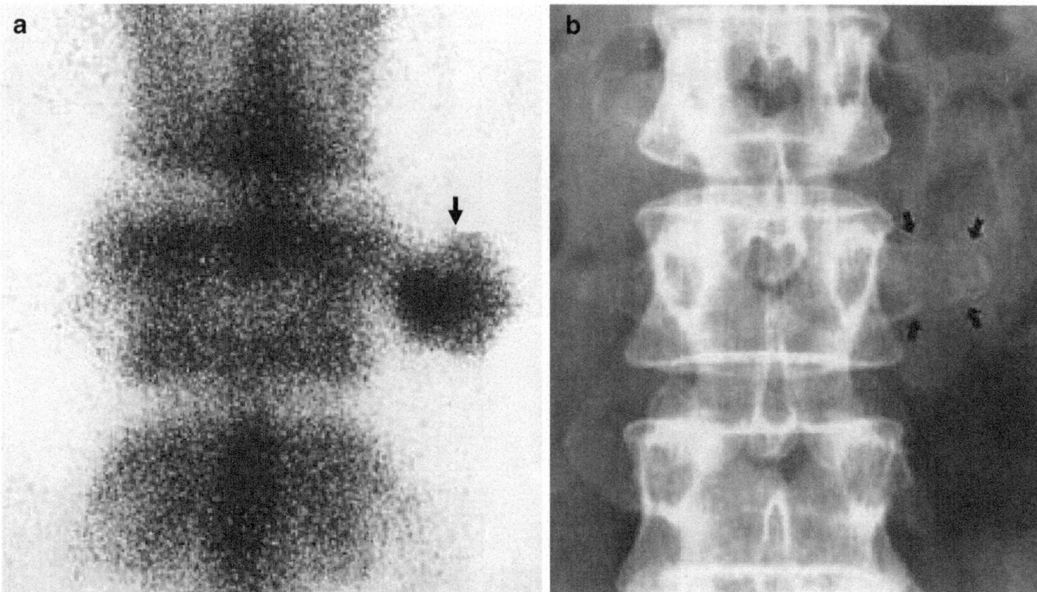

Fig. 2.4 Large anatomical structures can be snugly covered by the 10-cm field of view of pinhole scan. (**a**) For example, three life-size middle lumbar vertebrae can be included in adult showing malignant metastasis to the L3 left transverse process (arrow). (**b**) Conventional radiograph shows osteolysis in the L3 left transverse process (arrows)

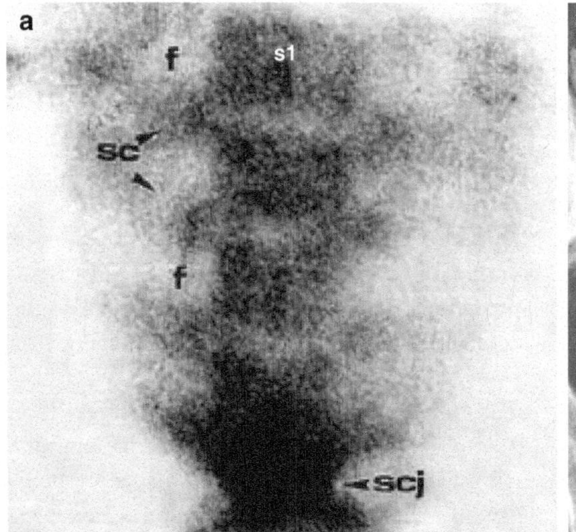

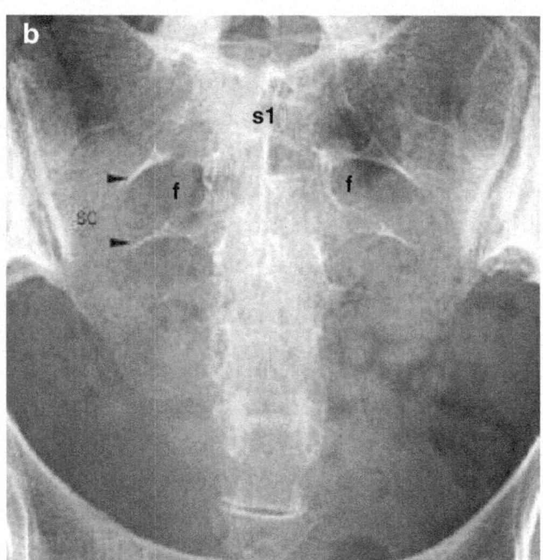

Fig. 2.5 Another example of one of the largest anatomical structures, the sacrum, well covered by a 10-cm field of view of pinhole scan. (**a**) One ^{99m}Tc-HDP pinhole scan can cover the whole sacrum including the sacroiliac joints, intervertebral foramina (f), sacral crest (sc), and sacrococcygeal articulation which is the common site of osteoarthritis with increased tracer uptake. (**b**) Conventional radiograph shows individual anatomy

to visualize 200-μm callused trabecular microfracture (Fig. 2.7). The diagnostic sensitivity of highly enhanced image quality of pinhole scan cannot be overemphasized. Indeed, parallel-hole bone scan shows only gross anatomy, but pinhole scan can reveal anatomy and pathological change in far greater detail (Figs. 2.1 and 2.2). It is not due to mere image size enlargement, but due to essentially different image resolution (Bahk 2017).

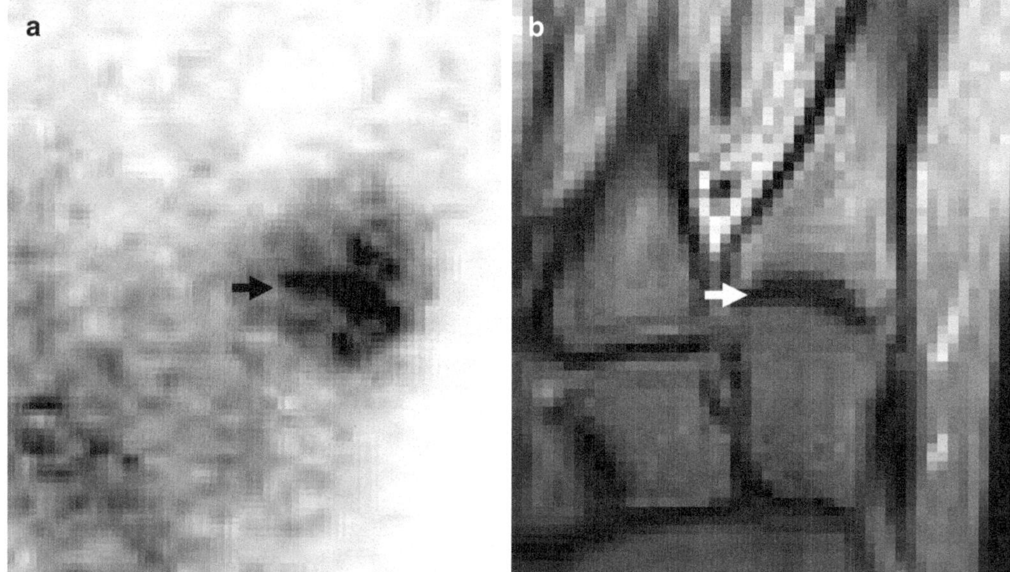

Fig. 2.6 Focal fracture in the base of the first metatarsal bone in a 20-year-old female. (**a**) Naïve pinhole scan shows blurry ^{99m}Tc-HDP uptake in the first metatarsal base fracture (arrow). (**b**) Axial T2-WT FS (3500/100) MR image shows a rod-like dark signal intensity in the first metatarsal bone base denoting fracture (arrow). This fracture is hard to distinguish on a radiograph because it was almost occult in nature

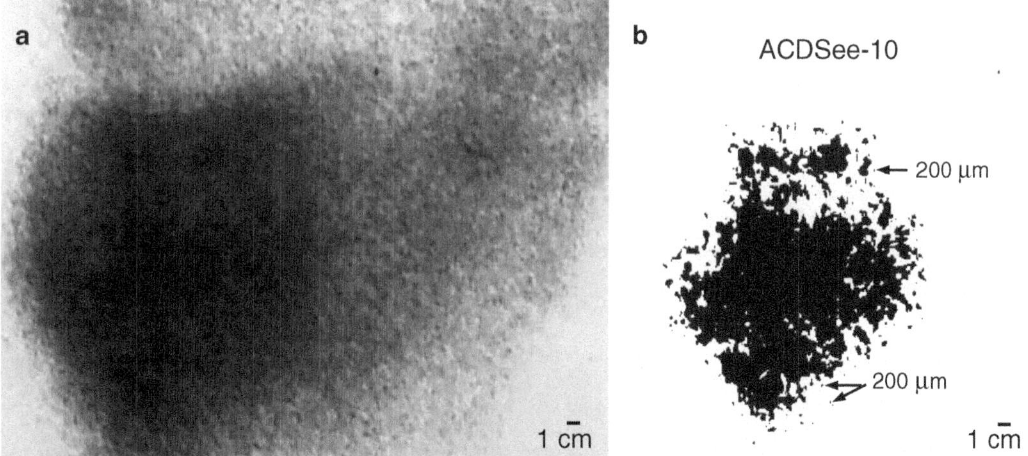

Fig. 2.7 Different demonstrations of numerous trabecular microfractures in the right lateral tibial condyle due to motor vehicle acccident using ACDSee-10 gamma correction pinhole scans in a 57-year-old male. (**a**) Naïve anterior ^{99m}Tc-HDP pinhole scan shows nonspecific blurry tracer uptake. (**b**) In contrast, gamma correction can neatly demonstrate a large central aggregated trabecular fractures and numerous microcalluses without penumbra. The smallest microcallus measures 200 µm in size

References

Bahk YW. Combined scintigraphic and radiographic diagnosis of bone and joint diseases with gamma correction interpretation. 5th ed. Heidelberg/Berlin: Springer; 2017.

Bahk YW, Kim OH, Chung SK. Pinhole collimator scintigraphy in differential diagnosis of metastasis, fracture, and infections of the spine. J Nucl Med. 1987;28:447–51.

Kim SH, Chung SK, Bahk YW, et al. Whole body and pinhole bone scintigraphic manifestations of Reiter's syndrome: distribution patterns and early and characteristic signs. Eur J Nucl Med. 1999;26:163–70.

Gamma Correction

3

Gamma correction is a nonlinear image processing algorithm to code and decode the luminance (gray) or tristimulus (color) values in a still image or video system for specific purposes (Holst 1998). The nonlinear equation of power-law expression is $Vout = Vin^{1/\gamma}$, where the input (Vin) and output ($Vout$) are nonnegative real values and γ denotes gamma value. According to Pyonton (2003), the equation can even be $Vout = Vin^{\gamma}$ in the simplest case. Technologically, the gamma correction of naïve ^{99m}Tc-HDP pinhole scan is readily accessible and easily performed without economical burden, yet it can specifically reveal characteristics and more often than not even pathognomonic findings. For gamma correction, we initially used the earlier version of ACDSee-7 Photo Editor, which was most recently shifted to upgraded ACDSee-10 version. The gamma value of individual pathological HDP uptake presented on naïve pinhole scan can be manually adjusted so that, for example, fibrovascular zone in osteoid osteoma (Fig. 3.1), bone cyst wall fracture (Fig. 3.2), edema–hemorrhage–trabecular micro fracture

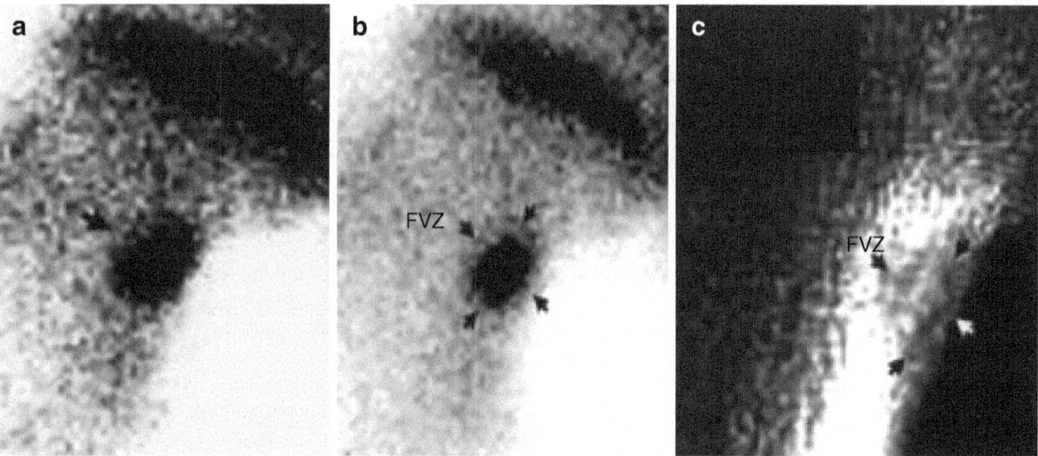

Fig. 3.1 Demonstration of nidus and fibrovascular zone (FVZ) in osteoid osteoma using gamma correction. (**a**) Naïve ^{99m}Tc-HDP pinhole scan of the right femoral neck in a 14-year-old male shows an ovoid lesion with intense uptake (arrow). (**b**) Gamma correction scan shows well-defined central nidus with intense tracer uptake and surrounding FVZ with lower tracer uptake (arrows). (**c**) Gamma correction radiograph (gamma = 12) shows calcified nidus and lucent FVZ (arrows)

Y.-W. Bahk, *Imaging of Trabecular Microfracture and Bone Marrow Edema and Hemorrhage*,
https://doi.org/10.1007/978-981-15-4466-8_3

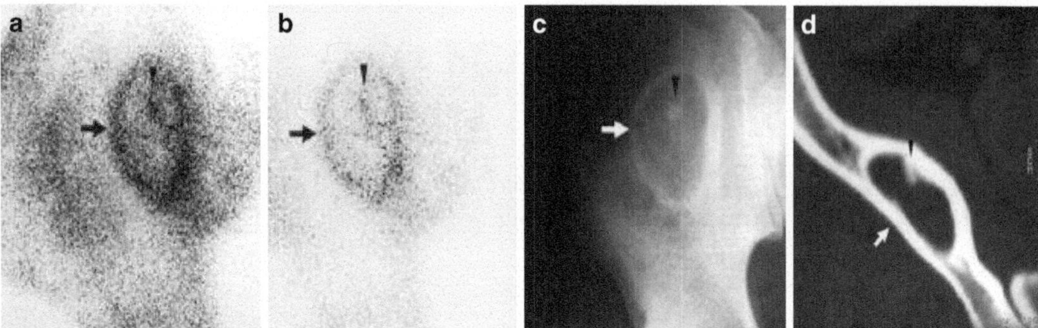

Fig. 3.2 Bone cyst in the flat right iliac bone in a 17-year-old male shows a large ovoid lucent lesion with spotty ^{99m}Tc-HDP uptake in the wall and an islet at 12 o'clock (arrowhead). (**a**) Anterior pinhole scan shows blurry tracer uptake (arrow). (**b**) Gamma correction view shows unsuppressed tracer uptake in the main cystic wall (arrow) and small islet uptake in upper half (arrowhead). (**c**) Anteroposterior radiograph shows cyst wall and an islet-like bone of undetached fracture (arrowhead). (**d**) Transaxial CT shows cyst with a thick wall (arrow) and an islet-like fracture arising from the anterior wall (arrowhead)

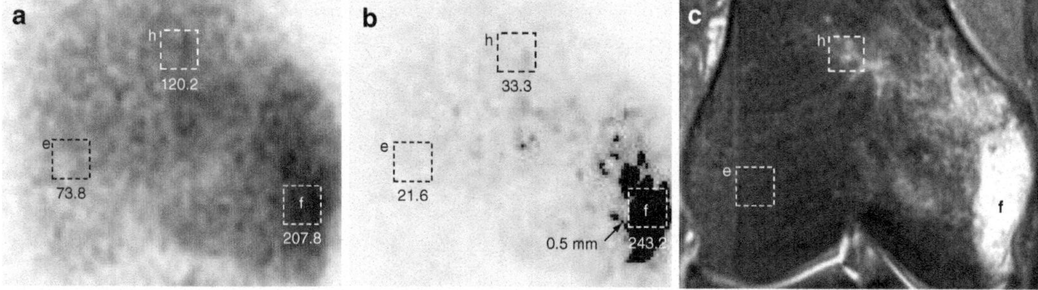

Fig. 3.3 Edema and hemorrhage can be differentiated using GCPBS and NIH ImageJ densitometry. This is an utmost simplified view to selectively pinpoint suppressed tracer uptake in edema and hemorrhage and highlighted uptake in fractures. (**a**) Naïve pinhole scan shows three 1-cm^2 areas of blurry tracer uptake of edema (*e*) and hemorrhage (*h*), and fracture (*f*) with the AU values being 73.8 in edema, 120.2 in hemorrhage, and 207.8 in fracture, respectively. (**b**) Typically, the gamma correction suppresses edema uptake down to AU = 21.6 and hemorrhage uptake down to AU = 33.3, but contrarily highlighting fractures (*f*) with significantly raised AU value to 243.2. The smallest fracture measures 500 μm in size. (**c**) Corroborative FS coronal T2-weighted MR image shows a 1-cm^2 area of hemorrhage (*h*) with bright signal intensity and another 1-cm^2 area of edema with little bright signal (*e*)

(Fig. 3.3), occult fracture (Fig. 3.4), cometary fracture with tail edema (Fig. 3.5), and callused trabecular microfracture (Fig. 3.6) can be specifically imaged and diagnosed. Additionally, the micron size of pinpointed callused TMF can be directly measured using the classic mathematic method (Jung et al. 2016) or a magnifying lens (Fig. 3.6). The usefulness of gamma correction in occult and cometary fractures is worthy of emphasis. Indeed, gamma correction pinhole bone scan is anticryptic in occult fracture (Fig. 3.4) and cometary fracture (Fig. 3.5). The gamma correction was first introduced to medial imaging in this monograph (Bahk 2013).

Gamma correction is an easily performed image processing algorithm of the Photo Correction Wizard program of an ACD Photo Editor. Currently, three versions are available in the market including ACDSee 7, ACDSee10, and ACDSee 22. Initially, we started our study using version 7 (Bahk et al. 2010; Jung et al. 2016) which was most recently shifted to upgraded version 10. It can cleanly suppress unfixed low tracer uptake in edema and moderate uptake in hemorrhage highlighting injured trabeculae with osteoneogenesis which accumulates high unsuppressed ^{99m}Tc-HDP (Bahk et al. 2017). We applied gamma correction to ^{99m}Tc-HDP pinhole bone scan to tentatively visualize callused TMF

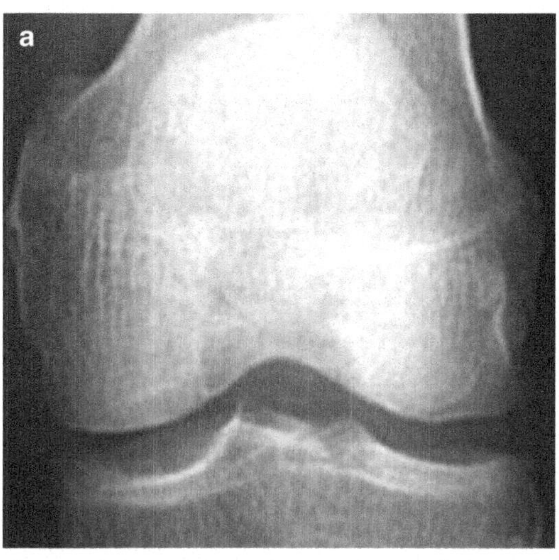

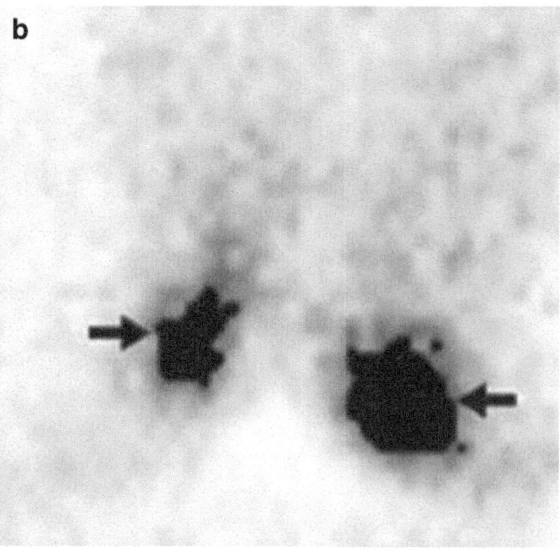

Fig. 3.4 Twin geographic occult fractures occurred in the left medial and lateral femoral condyles in a 53-year-old male. (**a**) Anteroposterior radiograph shows no abnormality. (**b**) However, gamma correction pinhole scan shows markedly increased ^{99m}Tc-HDP uptake in the fractures of the femoral condyles

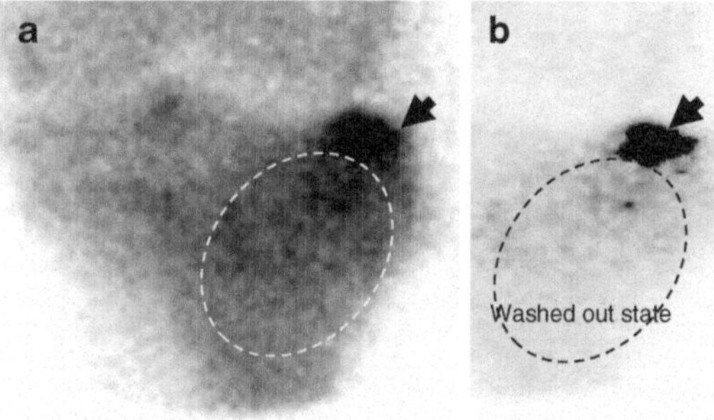

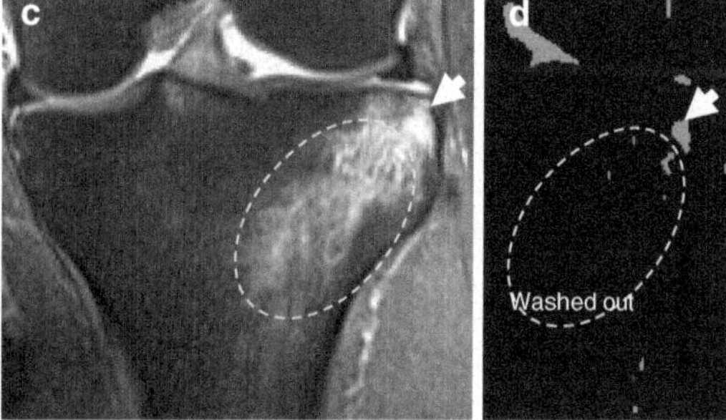

Fig. 3.5 Cometary fracture consists of the head fracture and tail edema with the fracture highlighted following the suppression of tail edema using gamma correction. (**a**) Naïve pinhole scan shows cometary fracture (arrow) with edematous tail (circle). (**b**) ACDSee-7 Gamma correction suppresses the edema uptake in the tail highlighting fracture with unsuppressed high tracer uptake (arrow). (**c**) Naïve coronal T2-weighted FS (3500/18) MR image shows a small geographic fracture in the tibial condyle with bright signal intensity (arrow) and edematous tail with gray signal intensity (circle). (**d**) Gamma correction washes out edema highlighting fracture with bright signal intensity in the condylar edge (arrow)

as unique in vivo imaging means and results thereof attained was clinically useful. Radiobiochemically, unsuppressed ^{99m}Tc-HDP uptake denotes actively ongoing osteoneogenesis. This monograph will primarily describe and discuss the refined use of the gamma correction pinhole bone scanning (GCPBS) in the diagnosis of most bone diseases including trabecular microfracture, osteoporosis, cervical sprain, whiplash injury, avascular necrosis, fish vertebra, sports injuries, osteitides, infection, benign and malignant neoplasms, and tumorous conditions (Bahk 2017). In particular, we attempted to differentiate edema and hemorrhage and trabecular microfracture from the standpoints of anatomical characterization and the quantification of ^{99m}Tc-HDP uptake profile. Furthermore, we made an attempt to extend gamma correction not only to MRI and CT but also to conventional radiography. The extended study was focused to further prove the usefulness of gamma correction in the imaging of CTMF (trabecular microfracture) which ubiquitously occurs in nearly all bone diseases. Imaging machines of MRI and CT and thereby attained images of trabeculae may differ according to

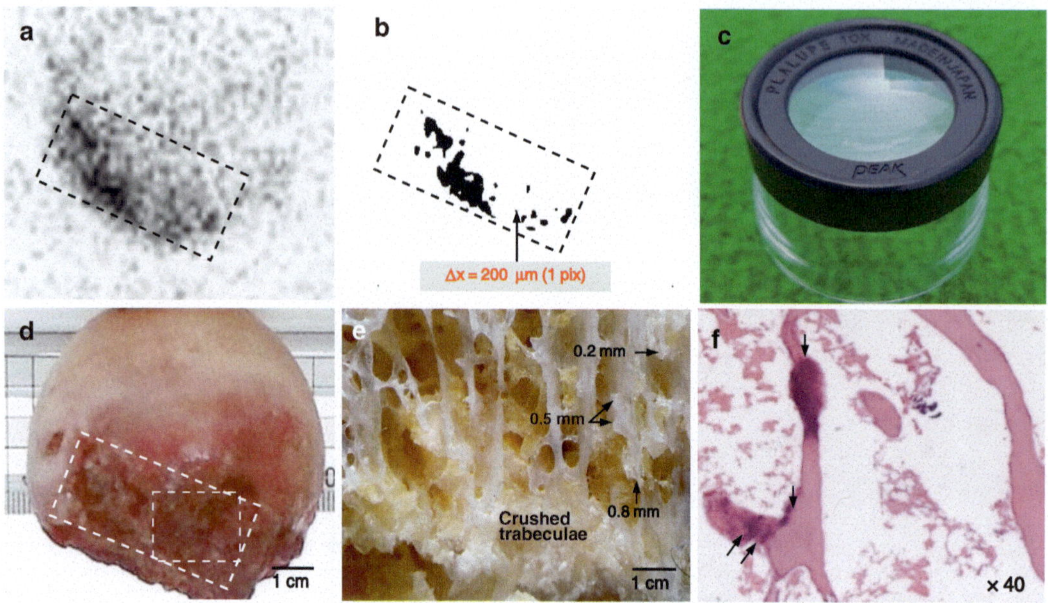

Fig. 3.6 Gamma correction pinhole scan demonstration and quantitation of 200 μm microcallus formed in trabecular fracture. (**a**) Naïve coronal ^{99m}Tc-HDP pinhole scan of operatively removed femoral head shows microfractures blurred due to edema and hemorrhage (frame). (**b**) Gamma correction scan highlights single pixel callused microfractures measured using 10× magnifying optic lens. Δx is x-axis. (**c**) Magnifying lens. (**d**) Surgical specimen shows irregular seed-pearly calluses. (**e**) Surface microscope shows callused seed-pearly microcalluses. (**f**) H&E stain shows typical base stained microcalluses and contused trabeculae with endosteal rimming. This case proves that microcallus is composed of pixel which can be precisely and handily quantitated using a magnifying optic lens

machine type and version. Generally, CR well retains its fine anatomical demonstrability of trabeculae but with unfortunate inborn inability to assess microtrabecular metabolism. Advantageously enough, gamma correction PBS can simultaneously achieve in vivo anatomical imaging and bone metabolic assay without difficulty. Indeed, it can manifest not only fine trabecular anatomy but also simultaneously provide bone metabolic profile which may differ from tissue to tissue (Figs. 3.1–3.3), and even efficiently differentiate bone marrow edema and hemorrhage and trabecular changes (Fig. 3.3). It is a unique imaging achievement reached in recent years (Bahk et al. 2019). Edema and hemorrhage and trabecular microfracture are well-known three basic pathological changes of bone marrow but until now they were out of our imaging diagnostic reach. Furthermore, it is of considerable imaging gain that the intricate pathological changes which occur in peri- and paraosseous tissues are fortuitously yet precisely observable. For example, the nidus and fibrovascular zone in osteoid osteoma can be selectively imaged and specifically diagnosed (Fig. 3.1) and bone cyst proper and rare complicating cystic wall fracture can likewise be precisely imaged and identified as such when the fracture fragment is vascularized (Fig. 3.2). In vivo diagnosis of such intricate pathological state appears not possible by any other imaging modalities at this time.

Trabecular microfracture heals by microcallus formation that surrounds trabeculae and a callused trabecular fracture measures approx. 500 μm in diameter in macerated cancellous bone slices (Vernon-Roberts and Pirie 1973). Lately, the callused microfracture became to be precisely imaged and measured using GCPBS which makes it distinctly highlighted by the suppression of disturbing blurry edema and hemorrhage tracer uptake. The smallest microcallus so demonstrated measured 200 μm in size in adults (Fig. 3.6; Bahk et al. 2017). As described, the suppression of ^{99m}T-HDP by gamma correction is considered to be related to its loose adhesion onto crystalline hydroxyapatite. Naturally, ^{99m}Tc-HDP uptake is not suppressed in actively growing bone physis and also in repair osteoneogenesis. A technical study designed and performed by us on the comparative efficacy of gamma correction in multiparallel hole collimator and pinhole collimator scans showed unquestionable superiority of the latter collimator in the diagnosis of fine bone pathology (Fig. 3.7e). Such a difference is considered to be due to the basically different finer image resolution and richer photon acquisition of ^{99m}Tc-HDP pinhole bone scan. Actually, the photon acquisition of pinhole scan is twice higher than that of parallel collimator scan as assessed by the measurement of photon acquisition in the knee bones in 30 cases. It is presumed to have resulted at least principally from the fact that pinhole scan is 3D volumetric gamma-ray imaging, whereas MRI and CT are 2D imaging. Conventional radiograph is a typical 3D image but peculiarly enough fracture is more often than not concealed and occult. The fact that the image of complex fractures on GCPBS is much better defined than that of multiple parallel hole collimator scan as shown in Fig. 3.7. It is also to be mentioned that the demonstrability of trabecular injury is by far distinct on pinhole bone scan compared to MRI, CT, and CR (Fig. 3.8). This difference may be explained on the basis of two facts: the high sensitivity and specificity of tracer uptake and the volume gain of radiotracer in 3D imaging (Fig. 3.8a). Conventional radiography is similarly benefitted by 3D imaging but the diagnostic specificity is not as high as pinhole scan (Fig. 3.8d). Our limited comparative study of pinhole scan, MRI, CT, and conventional radiograph showed that the most reliable single imaging diagnosis of CTMF (callused trabecular microfracture) can be made using gamma correction ^{99m}Tc-MDP pinhole bone scan. In particular, pinhole bone scan is able to uniquely demonstrate the fine anatomy of CTMF along with bone metabolic profile making it useful as a validation image to replace histopathology when demanded (Fig. 3.6b, e).

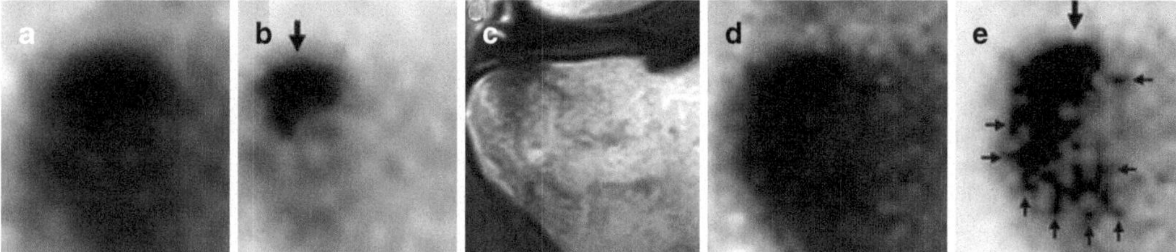

Fig. 3.7 Basically different arboriform fracture presentations in gamma correction multiparallel hole and gamma correction pinhole scans. (**a**, **b**) Pre- and post-gamma correction parallel hole scans of branching fracture in the lateral tibial condyle of the right tibia shows no branching at all. (**c**) Model T1-weighted MRI shows an arboriform branching fracture (arrow). (**d**) Naïve pinhole scan shows just nonspecific, homogeneous tracer uptake (arrow). (**e**) Amazingly, however, gamma correction view shows an arboriform fracture arising from a geographic base

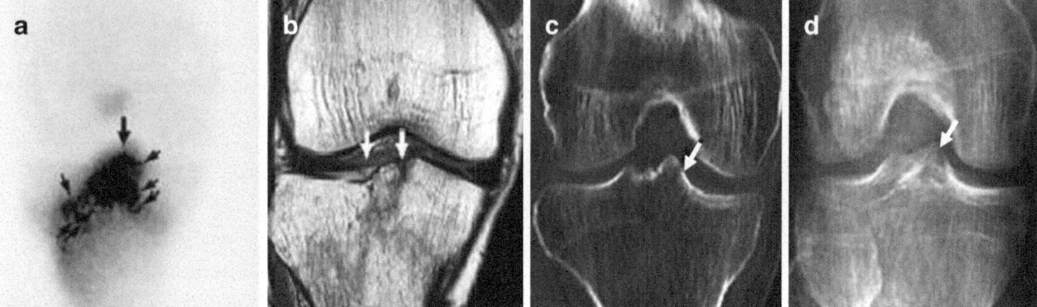

Fig. 3.8 Differential demonstrability of compound fractures by gamma correction of ^{99m}Tc-HDP pinhole scan, MRI, CT, and conventional radiography. (**a**) Gamma correction pinhole scan can most distinctly demonstrate fractures with impressive dark tracer uptake (arrows). (**b**) T2-weighted MRI shows several fractures with low signal intensity (arrows). (**c**, **d**) CT and radiographic demonstration are not so impressive. On the whole, fractures are most clearly demonstrated using ^{99m}Tc-HDP pinhole scanning. It is also true that gamma correction pinhole bone can unmistakably depict fracture as osteoneogenesis in acute callus does intensely accumulate ^{99m}Tc-HDP without failure

3.1 ACDSee Gamma Correction ^{99m}Tc-HDP Pinhole Bone Scan Diagnosis of Trabecular Microinjuries

We accidentally found that gamma correction can selectively suppress the mild to moderate blurry ^{99m}Tc-HDP uptake in bone marrow edema and hemorrhage distinctly highlighting CTMF which is characterized by unsuppressed tracer uptake. We used the phenomenon for the specific and differential diagnosis of CTMF in the rat (Bahk et al. 2016) and in human surgical specimens (Bahk et al. 2017) and for the differential diagnosis of bone marrow edema and hemorrhage and trabecular microfracture in human patients (Bahk et al. 2019).

Currently, three different versions of gamma correction are available in the market including ACDSee 7, ACDSee 10, and most lately ACDSee 22. ACDSee-7 was used in our earlier investigation and ACDSee 10 version is used in more recent studies. Basically, ACDSee gamma corrections are processed by clicking the toolbars on the monitor screen in the following sequence: exposure autoexposure to maximize uptake intensity done and save with a new name → exposure → image-brightness control by increasing gamma value to best visualize fracture → done and save with the finished image with another new name. Starting from 50 (the default value in Photo Editor) the gamma value is gradually increased until trabecular microfracture with intense ^{99m}Tc-HDP uptake is extracted following the suppression of loosely adherent but not chemically incorporated tracer in edema and congestion (Fig. 3.9). Gamma value is gradually increased until the faint ^{99m}Tc-HDP uptake in normal host bone (Fig. 3.10) and mild to moderate tracer uptake in edema and hemorrhage is suppressed leaving unsuppressed microfractures behind (Fig. 3.11). The gamma value so adjusted ranged from 70 to 95 depending on the quality of the naive original bone scan. Generally, pinhole scan with low tracer uptake needs lower gamma value increment and vice versa. It is to be remarked that higher tracer uptake naturally occurs in an actively growing bone physeal plates and also in reparative osteoneogenesis in callusoid endosteal rimming as incited by relatively mild bone contusion (Fig. 3.11). Contrarily, the gamma value is to be decreased down to 20 or less in MR image. The use of original naïve bone scans provided by the digital information and

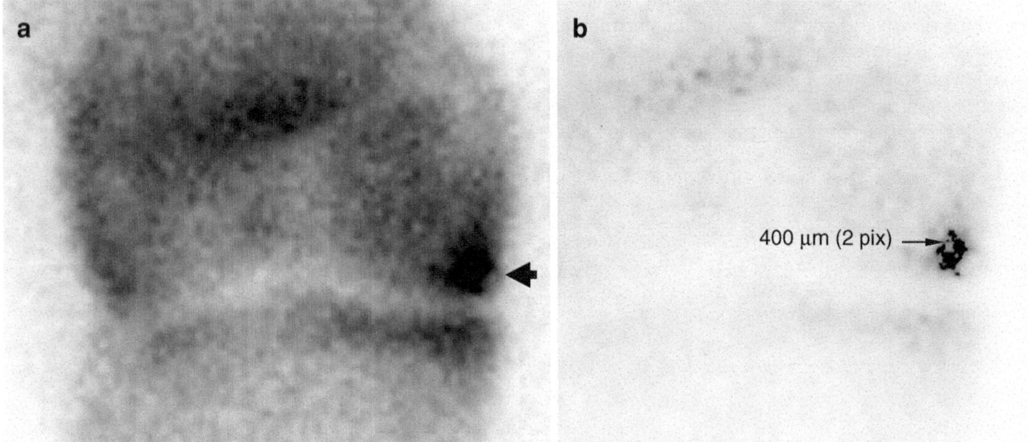

Fig. 3.9 Diffuse edema in the right medial femoral and tibial condyles with focal trabecular microfractures in the femoral condylar edge in a 54-year-old man due to falling into a manhole. Gradual increase in gamma value suppresses uptake edema highlighting callused trabecular fractures. (**a**) Naïve ^{99m}Tc-HDP pinhole bone scan demonstrates diffusely increased tracer uptake with a small mottled area of higher uptake in the medial femoral condylar edge (arrow). (**b**) ACDSee-7 gamma correction view shows the suppression of edema uptake disclosing microfractures in the medial femoral condylar edge. The smallest fracture measures 400 μm (2 pix) in size

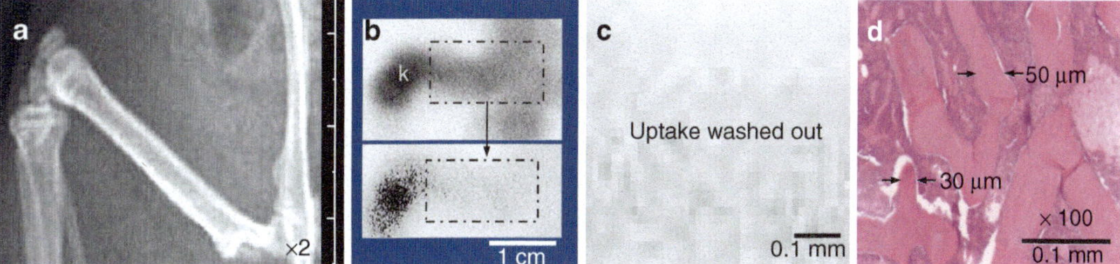

Fig. 3.10 Normal control femur in a young rat. (**a**) Twofold magnified radiograph shows no fracture or trabecular change. (**b**) Top frame is naïve normal rat ^{99m}Tc-HDP pinhole scan showing faint physiological tracer uptake (frame) and bottom frame shows clean suppression. (**c**) Magnified gamma correction view shows the complete suppression of faint tracer uptake. (**d**) H&E stain of normal trabeculae in young rat shows scarcely visible endosteum with the smallest one measuring 30 μm in thickness

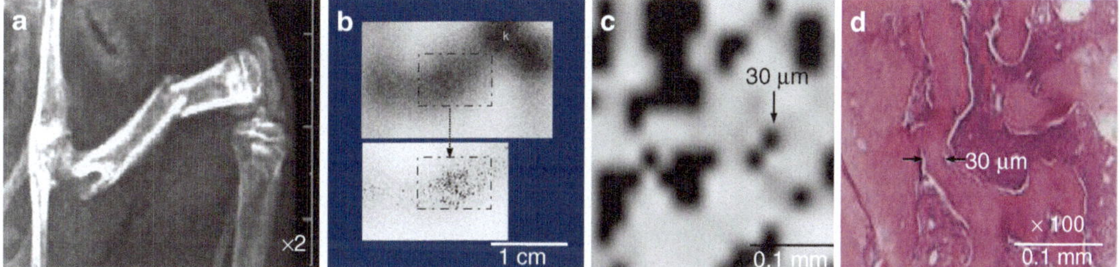

Fig. 3.11 Experimentally induced femoral shaft fracture and contusion in young rats. (**a**) Twofold magnified radiograph shows fracture and trabecular contusion which is occult. (**b**) Top frame: twofold magnified naïve pinhole scan shows nonspecific blurry increased tracer uptake (frame) and bottom frame shows suppression of edema and hemorrhage uptake presenting gamma correction microfractures which are too small to be seen with unaided eyes (frame). (**c**) ×50 magnified ACDSee-7 gamma correction view shows variously shaped trabeculae with unsuppressed intense tracer uptake due to endometrial rimming. The smallest one measures 30 μm in size. Observe blurry contour due to penumbra. (**d**) H&E stain distinctly shows endosteal rimming with the smallest one measuring 30 μm in thickness

communications in medicine (DICOM) without any modification is necessary. This precaution is important and when neglected gamma correction would end as useless. Our paired control study on the comparative efficacy of gamma correction in multiple parallel-hole collimator and pinhole collimator scan test showed that the latter is by far superior in image quality as anticipated (Fig. 3.7). Gamma correction is actually useless in multiple parallel-hole bone scan. Such a difference is theorized to be due to incomparably higher resolution and richer photon yielding of pinhole bone scan. The photon acquisition of a pinhole scan is twice larger than that of a parallel hole collimator scan as assayed by the measurement of photon acquisition in bones of the knee in 30 consecutive cases.

Sequentially, the procedures of image processing by ACDSee-10 are to be described here in detail. The naïve MR image is imported to ACDSee-10, and the "filter" in the top menu bar is selected. Then, select the "Exposure/Lighting" and "Exposure" again. There are three sliding bars to control: (1) Exposure, (2) Contrast, and (3) Fill Light. The default values in the control bar are all set to zeros. In our study, exposure and contrast were particularly enhanced in both MR image and pinhole scan presented in the black-and-white mode.

Lately, visuospatial-mathematic assay (VSMA) technique was developed by us (Bahk et al. 2019). It was purposefully designed and performed to differentiate acute bone marrow edema, bone marrow hemorrhage, and trabecular

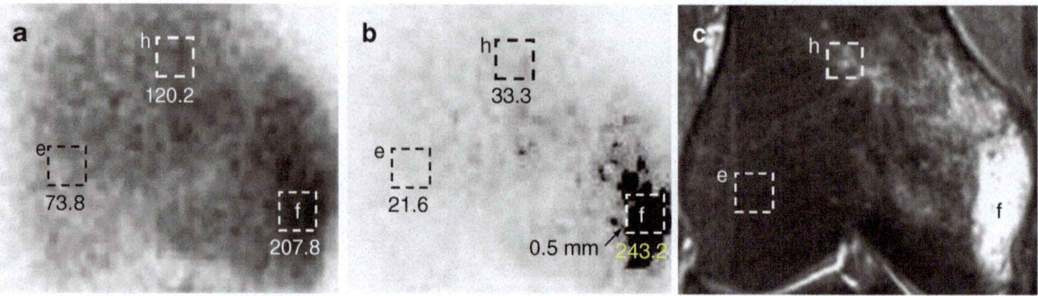

Fig. 3.12 Edema and hemorrhage can be differentiated using GCPBS and NIH ImageJ densitometry. This is an utmost simplified view to feature suppressed tracer uptake in edema and hemorrhage and highlighted uptake in fractures. (**a**) Naïve pinhole scan shows three 1-cm² areas of blurry tracer uptake of edema (*e*) and hemorrhage (*h*), and fracture (*f*) with the AU values being 73.8 in edema, 120.2 in hemorrhage, and 207.8 in fracture, respectively. (**b**) Gamma correction suppresses edema (AU = 21.6) and hemorrhage uptake (AU = 120.2) highlighting fractures (*f; AU* = 243.2). The smallest fracture measures 500 μm in size. (**c**) Corroborative FS coronal T2-weighted MR image (3,500/18) shows a 1-cm² area of hemorrhage (*h*) with bright signal intensity and another 1-cm² area of edema with little bright signal (*e*)

microfractures that have long been considered to be one of the toughest imaging tasks. VSMA can be done by triple use of: (1) seriated naïve and conventional gamma correction pinhole bone scans, (2) NIH ImageJ densitometry in terms of arbitrary units, and (3) pixelized measurement of microcallus size. The usefulness of this differential method was verified by the foregoing gold standard of gamma correction ^{99m}Tc-HDP pinhole bone scan findings as shown in Fig. 3.12. Using this tripple method, bone marrow edema and bone marrow hemorrhage and trabecular microcallus can be usefully differentiated. Technically, bone marrow edema was first differentiated from marrow hemorrhage and thereafter trabecular fractures were distinguished from edema and hemorrhage in sequence. Such distinction was based on the difference of NIH ImageJ densitometry value in terms of Arbitrary Unit.

^{99m}Tc-HDP pinhole bone scan, CT, and MRI have been continuously improved technically to advantageously respond to clinical demands. For instance, a bone scan is now more or less regularly taken using a pinhole collimator to refine the anatomical detail of bone scan along with specific bone metabolic information and such scan is further enhanced by gamma correction. Indeed, naïve PBS and GCPBS can be beneficially used for the differentiation and identification of bone marrow edema, hemorrhage, and trabecular microfracture which are unrecognizably intermixed. But three basic bone marrow changes can now be individually identified as such and differentiated one form the other using visuospatial-mathematic assay (VSMA) (Bahk et al. 2019). VSMA makes good use of ImageJ densitometry of NIH (http://rsb.info.nih.gov/ij) as shown in Fig. 3.12.

On the other hand, the image quality of MRI and CT has been also continually upgraded to meet ever increasing clinical demands by constructing higher Tesla MRI with renewed technical program and thinner slicing CT with a new technical menu to build micrographic imaging diagnostics. Figure 3.13a is T1WT (502/40) MR image of the left knee showing an overt crescent-like fracture in the lateral tibial condyle which was occult and unseen at all in radiograph (Fig. 3.14b). Incidentally, this particular case demonstrates multiple coarsened trabeculae in the femoral and tibial condyles. Trabeculae are dark in MR image and conversely bright or radiopaque in radiograph. Radiograph does not show fracture and hence it is occult in nature.

The manual processing of ACDSee gamma corrections is described in the intermediary column of Fig. 3.14. For example, one naive MRI is processed using ACDSee-10. First, the "filter" in the top menu bar is selected. Second,

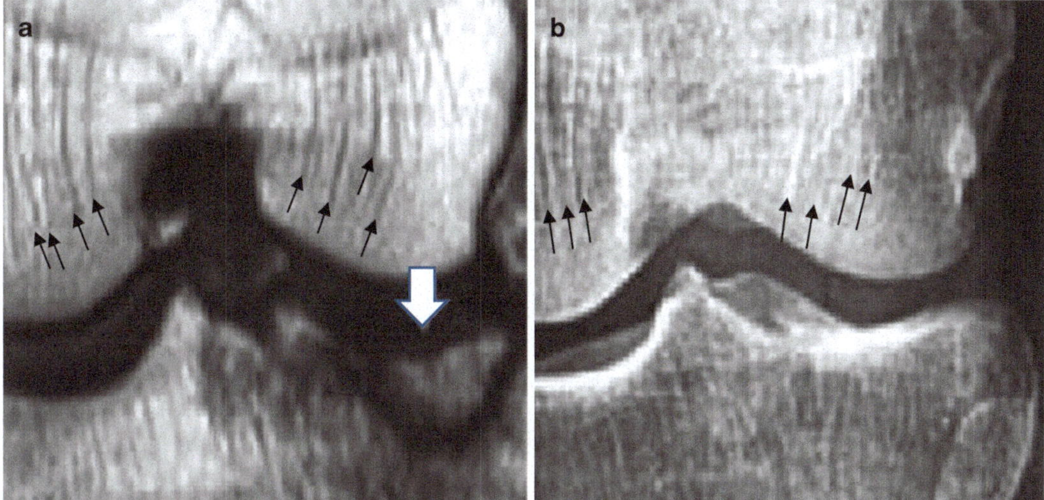

Fig. 3.13 Occult fracture in the left lateral tibial condyle and normal trabeculae in the apposing lateral femoral condyle in a 51-year-old woman. (**a**) T1WT (502/40) MR image of the left lateral tibial condyle shows prominent crescent fracture with dark signal intensity (large arrow) surrounded by blurry trabeculae. There are normal trabeculae in the apposing femoral condyles (smaller arrows). This MRI was taken using an old Signa Excite 1.5T, GE, Milwaukee, USA. (**b**) Conventional radiograph of the same patient shows no fracture or trabecular change. This is a typical occult fracture. Trabeculae are dark in MRI and bright in a radiograph

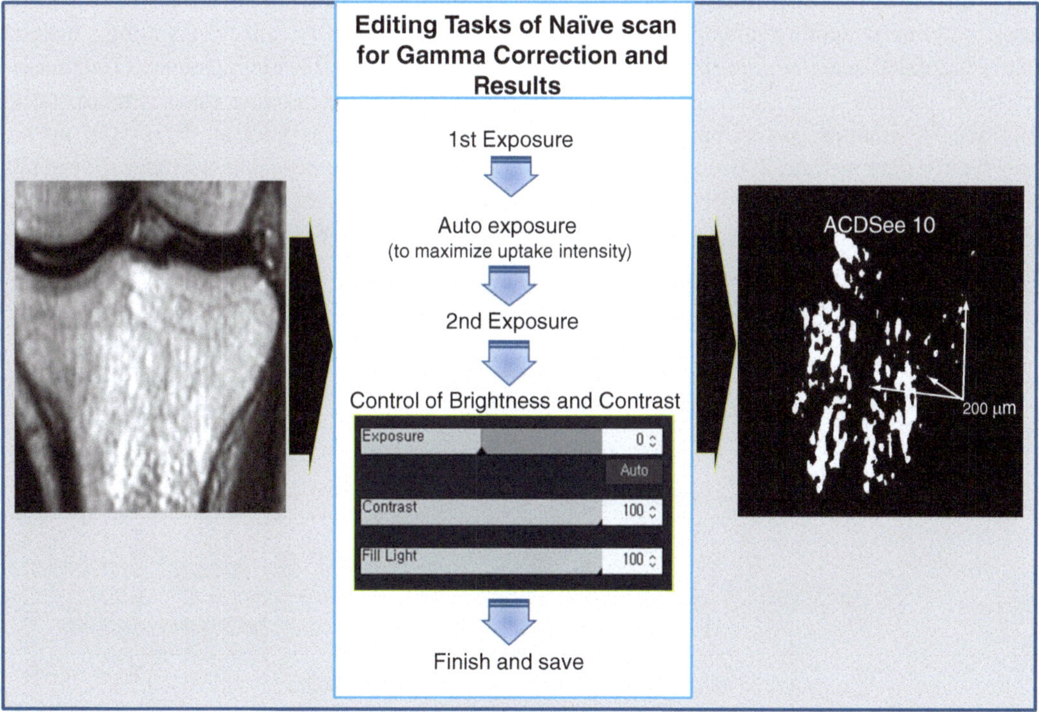

Fig. 3.14 Diagram of ACDsee 10 gamma correction procedures. Left column: naïve T2 WT (3500/85) FS coronal MR image shows numerous blurry nonspecific bright signal intensities incited by bicycle accident in a 78-year-old male. Intermediary column: editing tasks for gamma corrections. Right column: ACDSee-10 gamma correction view shows a great number of neatly defined mottled and pinpointed callused trabecular fractures including many 200-μm microfractures (arrows)

the "Exposure/Lighting" and "Exposure" are selected again. There are three sliding bars to control: (1) Exposure, (2) Contrast, and (3) Fill Light. Technically, default values in the control bar are all set to zero. In our study, exposure and contrast were particularly enhanced in MR image and ^{99m}Tc-HDP pinhole bone scan presented in the black-and-white mode. It is considered that the control of "exposure" provides the dynamic range of luminance in which we are interested and the control of contrast may amplify the perception of luminance in our eyes. After editing the image to optimally visualize microfracture the final image is saved with another new name. It is considered that the control of "exposure" provides the dynamic range of luminance in which we are interested and the control of contrast may amplify the perception of luminance in our eyes. Although we know only a little about what kind of technical changes were made in ACDSee 10 version resultant images showed neatly refined image quality of callused trabecular microfractures without penumbra along with significantly increased sensitivity to depict ATMF by upgraded gamma correction. It is true that ACDSee-10 gamma correction of MRI can very neatly demonstrate 200-μm callused trabecular microfracture without penumbra (Fig. 3.14).

3.2 ACDSee-10 Gamma Correction Pinhole Bone Scans

In order to specifically image CTMF ACDSee-7 was used in earlier phase but it was recently shifted to upgraded ACDSee-10. The purpose of the use of ACDSee gamma correction has remained unchanged and the same. It was and is used to specifically demonstrate CTMF by the suppression or removal of disturbing edema and hemorrhage in bone marrow injury. Gamma correction suppresses ^{99m}Tc-HDP which is loosely adhered to normal trabeculae in edema and hemorrhage highlighting the biochemically incorporated tracer in injured trabeculae. Technically, the naïve ^{99m}Tc-HDP pinhole scan of the surgically removed bone specimen was processed using the gamma correction of Photo Correction Wizard program of ACD Photo Editor of USA (ACDSee-10) to specifically demonstrate the characteristic ^{99m}Tc-HDP uptake in CTMF which measures 200 μm or unit pixel in size as imaged and measured by pixel counting method (Fig. 3.15). In performing gamma correction, as already explained, gamma value is increased to suppress the mild to moderate ^{99m}Tc-HDP uptake in normal and edema and hemorrhage dipped trabeculae to highlight CTMF with unsuppressed high tracer uptake. Once again, gamma correc-

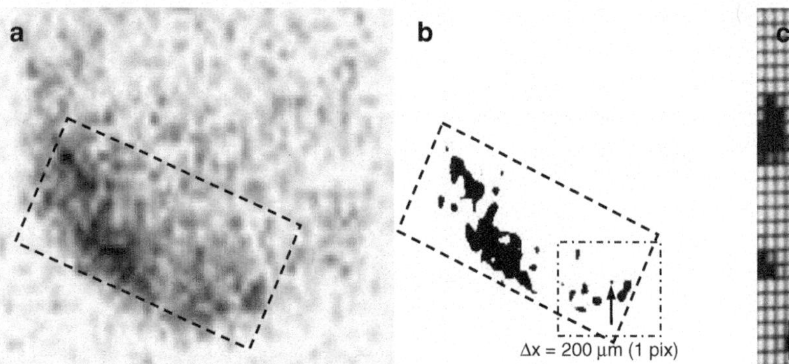

Fig. 3.15 Single unit pixel fracture involvement of ACDSee-10 gamma correction ^{99m}Tc-HDP pinhole bone scan imaged and quantified of 200 μm callused trabecular microfractures formed in the femoral neck fracture. (**a**) Naïve pinhole scan of the right femoral neck fracture shows non-specific blurry tracer uptake in microfractures due to edema and hemorrhage (*frame*). (**b**) Gamma correction highlights single pixel 200 μm microcallus. Δx is x axis. (**c**) Close-up view of single pixel microcallus taken using the built-in camera in cell phone (Galaxy Note 8, Samsung, Seoul)

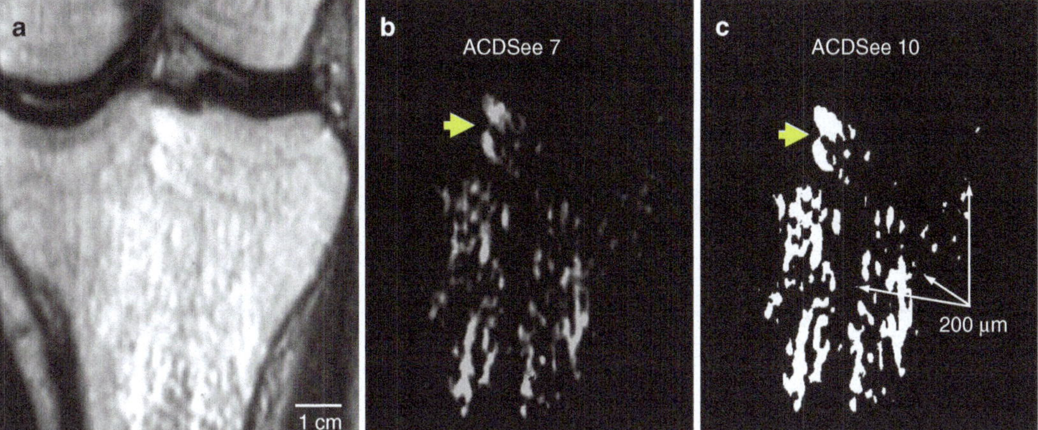

Fig. 3.16 Obvious difference of ACDSee 7 and ACDSee 10 gamma correction demonstrations of microcalluses in the right tibial tuberosity microcalluses incited by bicycle accident in a 78-year-old male. (**a**) Naïve T2 weighted (3,500/85) FS coronal MR image shows numerous non-specific blurry bright signal intensities. (**b**) ACDSee-7 gamma correction MR image shows incompletely suppressed blurry microcalluses due to penumbra (yellow arrow). (**c**) In contrast, however, ACDSee-10 gamma correction (−100/−71/−37) can neatly highlight archipelagic and micrometric callused trabecular microcalluses (yellow arrow). Additionally, upgraded gamma correction can sensitively demonstrate 200-μm microfractures (small arrows) which are not shown on ACDSee 7 gamma correction

tion is processed by clicking the toolbars in the following sequence: exposure and autoexposure to maximize uptake intensity and done and save with a new name. Then, exposure and image-brightness control are done by increasing gamma value up to 95 from 50 (the default value) and done and save the finished image with another new name. We found that ACDSee-10 is superior both in image resolution and in lesion demonstrability (sensitivity) than ACDSee 7 (Fig. 3.16).

3.3 Difference Between ACDSee 7 and ACDSee-10 Gamma ^{99m}Tc-HDP Pinhole Bone Scans

The principle and processing of ACDSee 10 are considered to be basically the same as those of ACDSee-7 gamma correction but end results are much different. It is processed by clicking toolbars on the monitor screen in the following sequence as described in Sect. 3.1. Gamma value is increased up to 95 or more until trabecular microcallus in microfracture is highlighted following the suppression of edema and congestion uptake (Fig. 3.17). Usually, so adjusted gamma value ranges from 70 to 95 depending on the quality of the naive bone scan. Generally, pinhole scan with a low tracer uptake needs low gamma value increment and vice versa. It is to be noted that high tracer uptake occurs in growing physis (Fig. 3.18), callusoid endosteal rimming (Fig. 3.19), CTMF (Fig. 3.20), and malignant bone metastasis (Fig. 3.21).

By surgical specimen analysis, we were able to confirm that ACDSee-10 gamma correction is superior to ACDSe-7 neatly eliminating penumbra and enhancing diagnostic sensitivity of CTMF (Fig. 3.16). We noted that the unsuppressed ^{99m}Tc-HDP uptake in endosteal rimming (Fig. 3.19c), trabecular microcallus (Fig. 3.20b), and metastatic cancer (Fig. 3.21) are similar without differential features although there are two possible differential features. The one is the presence of fairly large archipelagic lesion of crushed trabeculae without history of trauma and the other one is lesion plurality and irregularity of bone destruction (Fig. 3.21). Conventional radiography shows osteolysis and osteosclerosis in combination. This interesting finding would need a future systematic investigation.

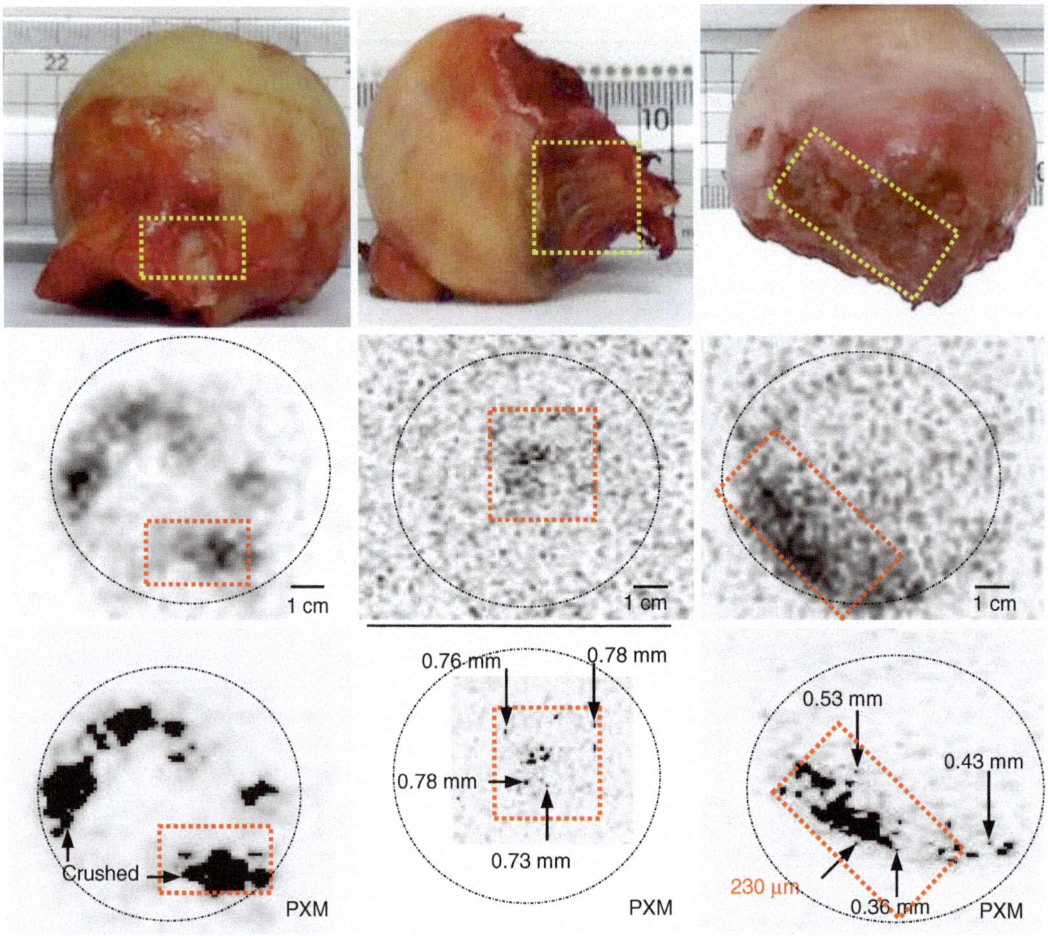

Fig. 3.17 Fresh surgical specimens, naïve pinhole scans, and gamma correction pinhole scans. Top panel: three different specimens show neck fracture surface with roughened bones including poorly defined calluses (frame). Intermediary panel: Naïve pinhole scans show blurry injured bones due to edema and hemorrhage. Bottom panel: ACDSee-7 gamma correction ^{99m}Tc-HDP pinhole scans show suppression of edema and hemorrhage distinctly highlighting pinpointed and crushed microcalluses. The smallest one measures 230 μm. PXM is pixelized measurement

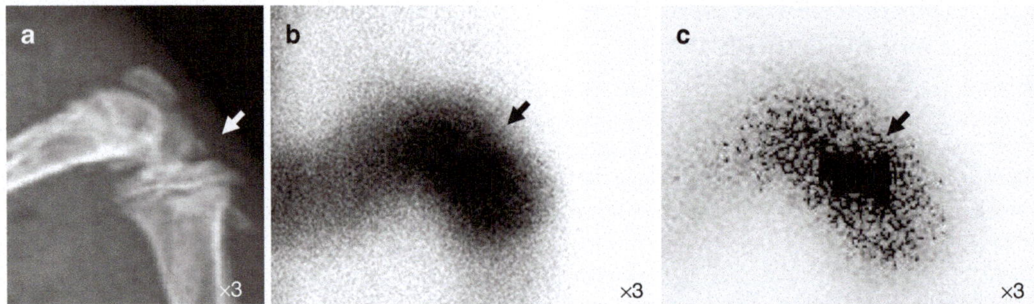

Fig. 3.18 Physiological intense tracer uptake in actively growing femoral and tibial physis in young rats. (**a**) Threefold enlarged radiograph shows open physeal lines (arrow). (**b**) Naïve pinhole scan shows intense tracer uptake in physeal zones (arrow). (**c**) Gamma correction view shows unsuppressed geographic tracer uptake in physes surrounded by numerous trabecular micro uptake in metaphyseal bones, the growth of which is considered to be gradually slowing down

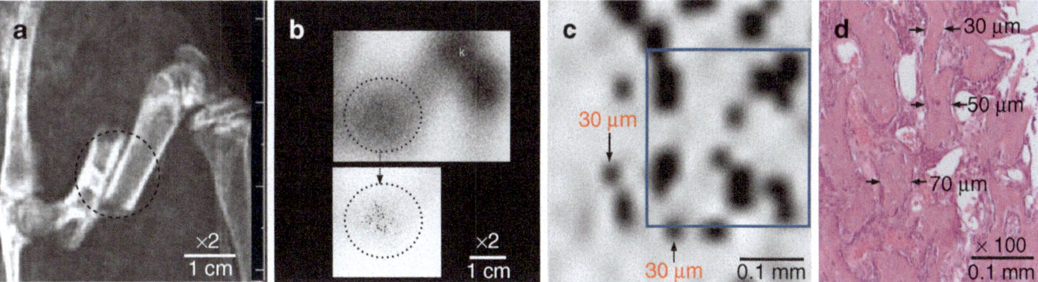

Fig. 3.19 Experimental endosteal rimming incited by a falling iron-ball hemorrhagic contusion in young rats. (**a**) Freely falling iron-ball induced fracture is shown but no microfractures are shown (circle). (**b**) Twofold magnified pinhole scan shows the hypocenter of trauma (circle). Top frame is naive scan and bottom frame is gamma correction view. (**c**) Magnified view of gamma correction PBS shows unsuppressed tracer uptake in trabecular endosteal rimming. (**d**) H&E stain (×100) shows endosteal rimming and diffuse hemorrhage

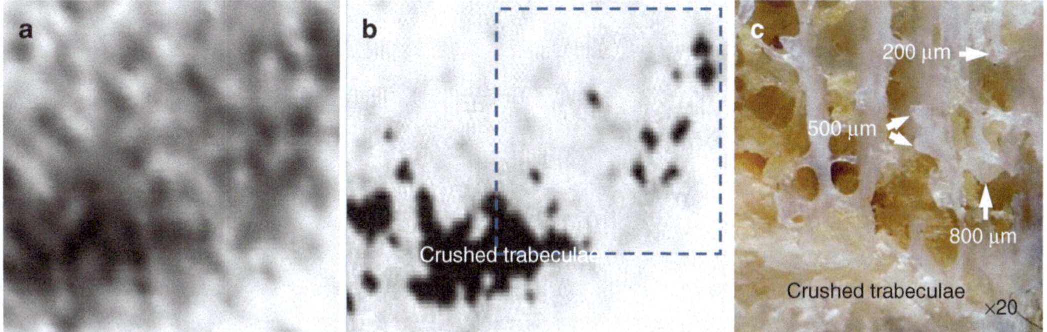

Fig. 3.20 Conventional ACDSee-7 gamma correction pinhole scan shows microcalluses and archipelagic crushed trabeculae in the femoral head removed for bipolar prosthesis in a 72-year-old female patient. (**a**) Naïve ^{99m}Tc-HDP pinhole scan shows nonspecific blurry tracer uptake. (**b**) ACDSee-7 gamma correction pinhole scan shows microcalluses and archipelagic fractures. ROI is framed. (**c**) Surface microscope of ROI in surgical specimen shows seed-pearly trabecular microfractures and large crushed trabeculae in the bottom

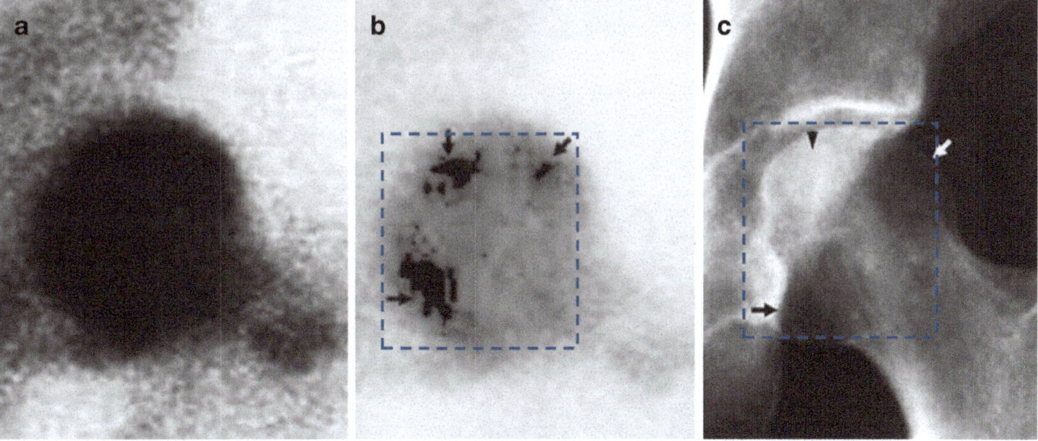

Fig. 3.21 Remarkable suppression of intense ^{99m}Tc-HDP in edema and hemorrhage from breast cancer metastasis in the left femoral head in a 41-year-old female. (**a**) Naïve ^{99m}Tc-HDP pinhole scan shows intense nonspecific blurry tracer uptake. (**b**) ACDSee-7 gamma correction pinhole scan shows dramatic suppression of edema and hemorrhage highlighting microcalluses and archipelagic fractures (frame). (**c**) Anteroposterior radiograph shows two poorly defined osteolysis (arrows) and osteosclerosis (arrowhead) suggesting metastases

References

Bahk YW, Jeon HS, Kim JM, et al. Novel use of gamma correction for precise (99m)Tc-HDP pinhole bone scan diagnosis and classification of knee occult fractures. Skeletal Radiol. 2010;39:807–13.

Bahk YW. Combined scintigraphic and radiographic diagnosis of bone and joint diseases with gamma correction interpretation. 4th ed. Heidelberg/Berlin: Springer; 2013.

Bahk YW. Combined scintigraphic and radiographic diagnosis of bone and joint diseases with gamma correction interpretation. 5th ed. Heidelberg/Berlin: Springer; 2017.

Bahk YW, Chung YA, Lee UY, Park SI. Gamma correction ^{99m}Tc-hydroxymethylene diphosphonate pinhole bone scan diagnosis and histopathological verification of trabecular contusion in young rats. Nucl Med Commun. 2016;37:988–91.

Bahk YW, Hwang SH, Lee UY, et al. Morphobiochemical diagnosis of acute trabecular microfractures using gamma correction Tc-99m HDP pinhole bone scan with histopathological verification. Medicine. 2017;96(45):e8419.

Bahk YW, Kim EE, Chung YA, et al. Precise differential diagnosis of acute bone marrow edema and hemorrhage and trabecular microfractrures using naïve and gamma correction pinhole bone scans. J Int Med Res. 2019; https://doi.org/10.1177/0300060518819910.

Holst GC. CCD arrays, cameras and displays. SPIE Optical Engineering Press, Bellingham: 1998. pp 169–171.

Jung J-Y, Cheon GJ, Lee Y-S, et al. Pixelized measurement of ^{99m}Tc-HDP micro particles formed in gamma correction phantom pinhole scan: a reference study. Nucl Med Mol Imaging. 2016;50:207–12.

Pyonton CA. Digital video and HDTV: algorithms and interfaces. Burlington: Morgan Kaufmann; 2003. pp. 260 and 630.

Vernon-Roberts B, Pirie CJ. Healing trabecular microfractures in the bodies of lumbar vertebrae. Ann Rheum Dis. 1973;32:406–12.

4 Gamma Correction ^{99m}Tc-HDP Pinhole Bone Scan of Trabecular Microfracture and Endosteal Rimming in Rat

During the recent years, we published some articles on gamma correction medical imaging, gamma correction ^{99m}Tc-HDP pinhole bone scan (GCPBS) in particular, for the specific diagnosis of callused trabecular microfracture (CTMF), bone contusion, and bone marrow edema and hemorrhage (Bahk et al. 2010, 2016, 2017, 2019). Those studies showed that the high ^{99m}Tc-HDP uptake in contused trabeculae is not suppressed by gamma correction, but the low uptake in intact bone trabeculae and edema and the moderate uptake in hemorrhage was cleanly suppressed. Originally, Francis et al. (1980) noted in their Sprague-Dawley rat experiment that ^{99m}Tc-HDP uptake was significantly increased in injured trabeculae because bone tracer was actively adsorbed onto amorphous calcium phosphate, which is actively engaged with osteoneogenesis in osteoblastic rimming of contused trabeculae. It was also shown that the nominal tracer uptake in intact bone and mild to moderate tracer uptake in bone edema and hemorrhage is due to loose adhesion of tracer onto crystalline hydroxyapatite. Recently, we also performed young rat experiment and confirmed the fact that the nominal tracer uptake in the normal trabeculae and mild to moderate tracer uptake (Fig. 4.1) in edema and hemorrhage are all cleanly suppressed by gamma correction, but the high uptake in CTMF is not suppressed at all (Fig. 4.2) (Bahk et al. 2016). To be exact the normal control study showed that the intact femur uniformly accumulates mild tracer, which is neatly suppressed by gamma correction barely showing endosteum on H&E stain (Fig. 4.1). Contrary, however, when trabeculae are well defined after gamma correction it may well denote that endosteal rimming is formed (Fig. 4.2). Unsuppressed high tracer uptake in epiphysis indicates that the physis in young rats is actively engaged with physiologically growing osteoneogenesis. The same biophysical phenomenon can be seen in CTMF, which is similarly engaged with active repair osteoneogenesis. It can be said that distinctly defined trabeculae may well be interpreted to designate endosteal rimming (Fig. 4.2).

We performed an experimental study in six young rats, one control and five traumatized, to histopathologically confirm and verify the suppression of micro ^{99m}Tc-HDP uptake in edema and/or hemorrhage irritated trabeculae (Bahk et al. 2016). Rats were a 3-week-old young male weighing 400–600 g and their bone injuries were considered to rapidly heal. Each rat was anesthetized using 5% isoflurane in 70% nitrous oxide and 30% oxygen in an induction chamber and anesthesia was maintained with a mixture of 2% isoflurane under temperature-controlled conditions (37 ± 0.1 °C) using a rectal thermometer and a heating pad. Rats were securely fastened to

Y.-W. Bahk, *Imaging of Trabecular Microfracture and Bone Marrow Edema and Hemorrhage*, https://doi.org/10.1007/978-981-15-4466-8_4

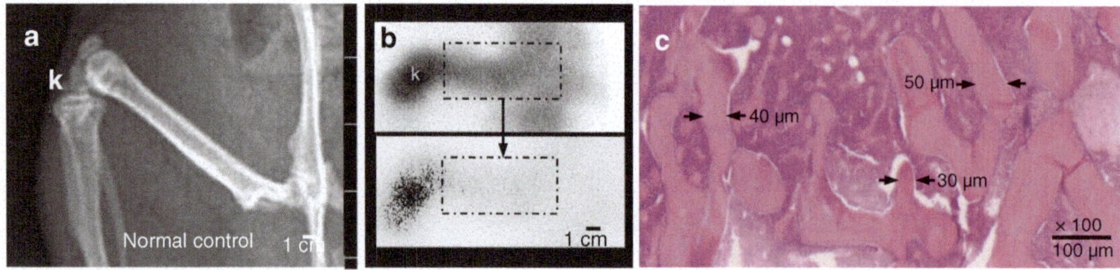

Fig. 4.1 Normal control 30-week-old young rat. (**a**) Radiograph of a normal control rat with 1-cm scale. The knee shows actively growing physes (*k*). (**b**) Top frame: rat pinhole scan shows intact femur with physiological tracer uptake in the growing knee bones (*k*) and low normal tracer uptake in the femoral shaft (*frame*). Bottom frame: animal pinhole scan shows clear suppression of normal femoral shaft uptake. (**c**) H&E stain shows normal trabeculae with scarcely visible intact endosteums (*arrows*)

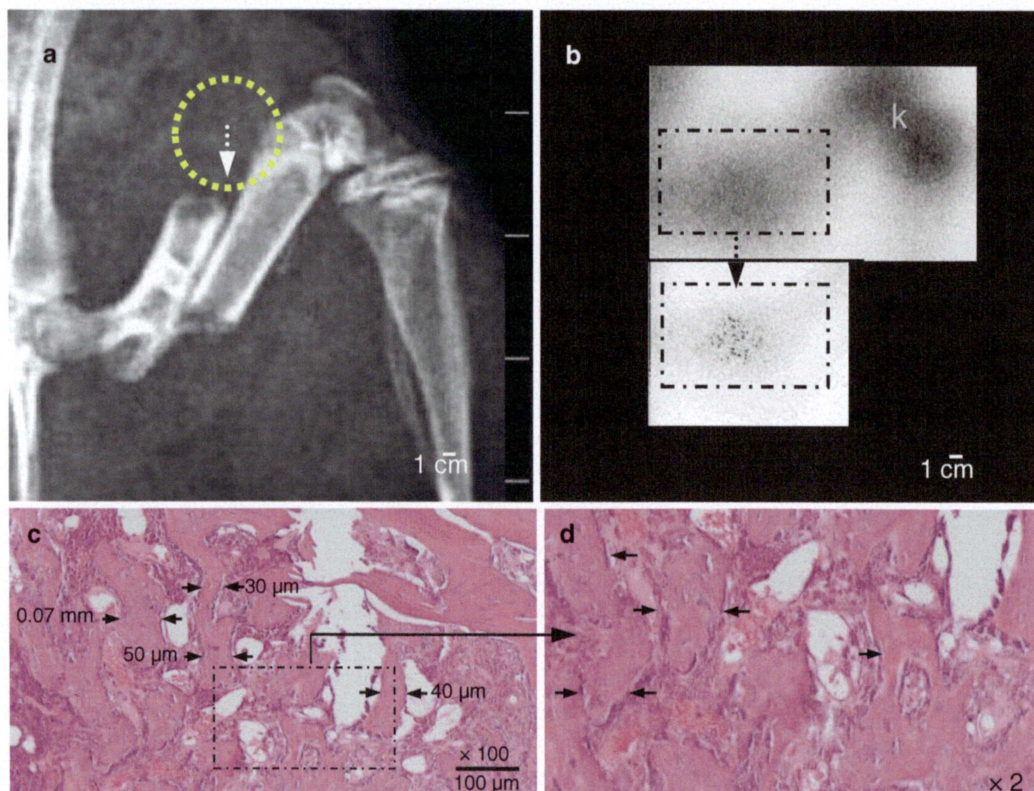

Fig. 4.2 Rat # 4 (30-week-old) shows fracture with fragment contraction in the middle shaft of the femur. (**a**) Radiograph shows a fracture with marked contraction (*arrow*). The knee shows actively growing physes. (**b**) Top frame: Naïve animal pinhole scan shows increased ^{99m}Tc-HDP uptake in the middle femoral shaft (*frame*) and high tracer uptake in growing knee bones (*k*) and low tracer uptake in the femoral shaft fracture (*frame*) and bottom frame shows unsuppressed tracer uptake in microfractures in trauma hypocenter. (**c**) H&E stain shows variously sized trabecular microfractures with callus formation and endosteal rimming. (**d**) Two-fold magnified view of framed portion of c clearly demonstrate endosteal rimming (arrows), hemorrhage, and microfractures

a stereotaxic apparatus and trabecular injury was inflicted on the right femoral shaft by means of blow impact from free-falling iron ball. Iron ball diameter was 2 cm and weight was 200 g. It was freely dropped from a height of 1 m (energy = 196 J) (Gläser et al. 2011)

4.1 Conventional Radiograph of Traumatized Young Rats

Six rats, one control and five fractured, underwent conventional radiography of the right femur 4 days post injury using automated exposure controls. Each radiograph with a metric scale was taken using model R-630-150 radiographic machine with 2-mm focal spot (Goldmountain, Songnam, South Korea). Figure 4.3 shows one normal control and five fractured rats.

4.2 Naïve and ACDSee-7 Gamma Correction ^{99m}Tc-HDP Pinhole Bone Scans Using Animal Bone Scanner in Young Rats

The femurs of one normal control rat and five test rats underwent ^{99m}Tc-HDP pinhole bone scanning using an animal scanner equipped with a 4-mm aperture pinhole collimator (Discovery NM630; GE Health care, Waukesha, Wisconsin, USA). The scans were performed 3 h after intravenous administration of 40.7 ± 1.48 MBq (1.1 ± 0.04 mCi) of ^{99m}Tc-HDP. Technically, the radioactivity of 220 kilocounts was accumulated. The original ^{99m}Tc-HDP pinhole bone scan image of the traumatized rat femur was too small to observe in its original size (Fig. 4.4).

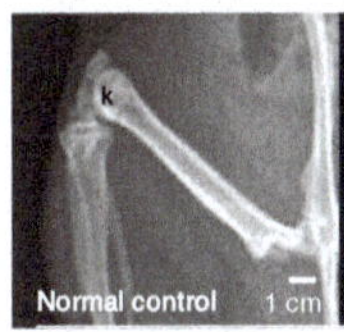

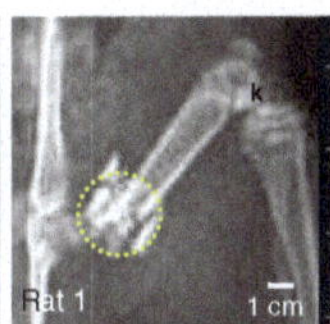

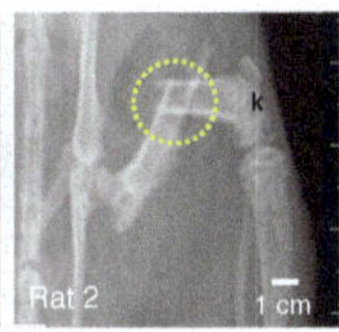

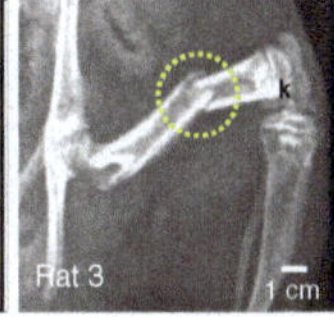

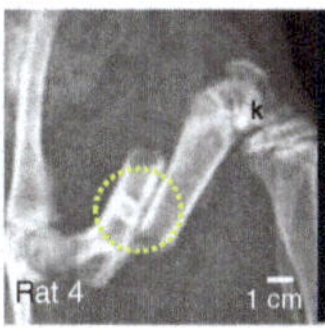

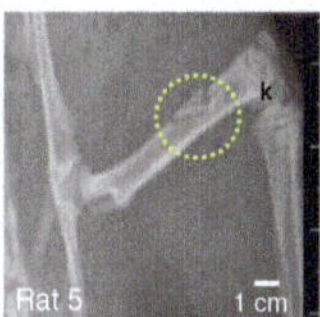

Fig. 4.3 All six rats, one normal control rat and five fractured rats, underwent conventional radiography of the right femur 4 days post injury using automated exposure controls. Each radiograph with a metric scale was taken using model R-630-150 radiographic machine with 2-mm focal spot (Gold-mountain Co., Songnam, South Korea). k is the knee. Hypocenters are marked with a circle

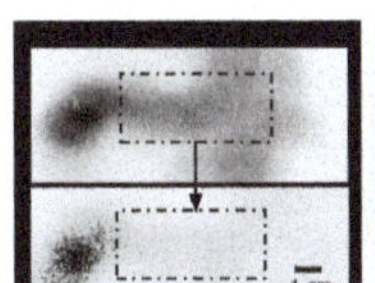

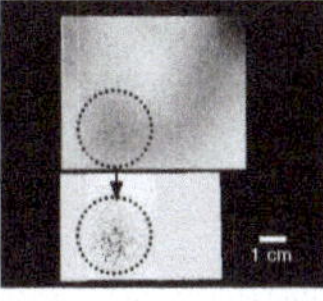

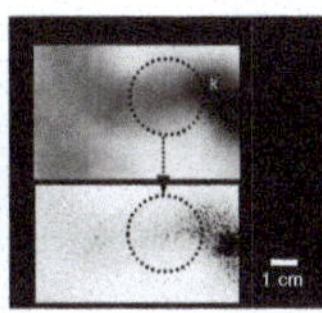

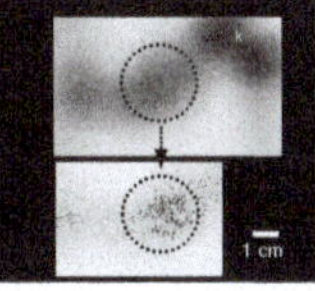

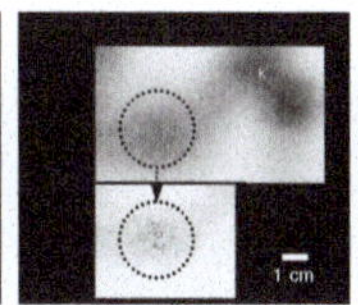

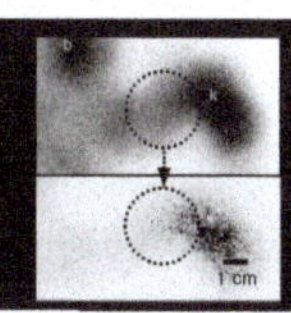

Fig. 4.4 One normal control young rat is presented in the first frame. It shows mild nominal physiological ^{99m}Tc-HDP uptake in the intact femoral shaft (frame) with intense tracer uptake in physeal ossification centers in the knee. In contrast, the injured femoral shafts of five rats show a focal area of increased tracer uptake in the hypocenter of falling iron-ball blow in the femoral shaft (circle). As shown in these cases actual pathological tracer uptake is extremely small in size needing appropriate magnification for image analysis and size assessment as will be seen in Fig. 4.8.

4.3 Gamma Correction ^{99m}Tc-HDP Pinhole Bone Scan and its 50-Fold Magnification View in Young Rats

Gamma correction was processed in the following manner (Bahk et al. 2010). First, "exposure" and "auto-exposure" were clicked to maximize uptake intensity and the image was saved with a new name. Second, "exposure" and "image brightness" were clicked and adjusted by increasing gamma value to neatly suppress lower uptake. Third and finally, "done" and "save" were clicked to finish the processing with another new name. The gamma value was increased from 50 (default value) to 95. Digital information and communication in medicine image (DICOM) were used without modification. As unsuppressed individual pathological ^{99m}TC-HDP uptake in naive GCPBS was small to see with unaided eyes, 1-cm ROI in the trauma hypocenter was electronically 50-fold magnified size assessment (Fig. 4.5).

4.4 Assessment of Gamma Correction ^{99m}Tc-HDP Pinhole Bone Scan Findings and Thereof Correlation with H&E Stain

The five traumatized rats were sacrificed 4 days after traumatization by intravenous injection of an overdose of urethane, and the femur was fixed for 24 h at 4 °C in 10% phosphate-buffered for-

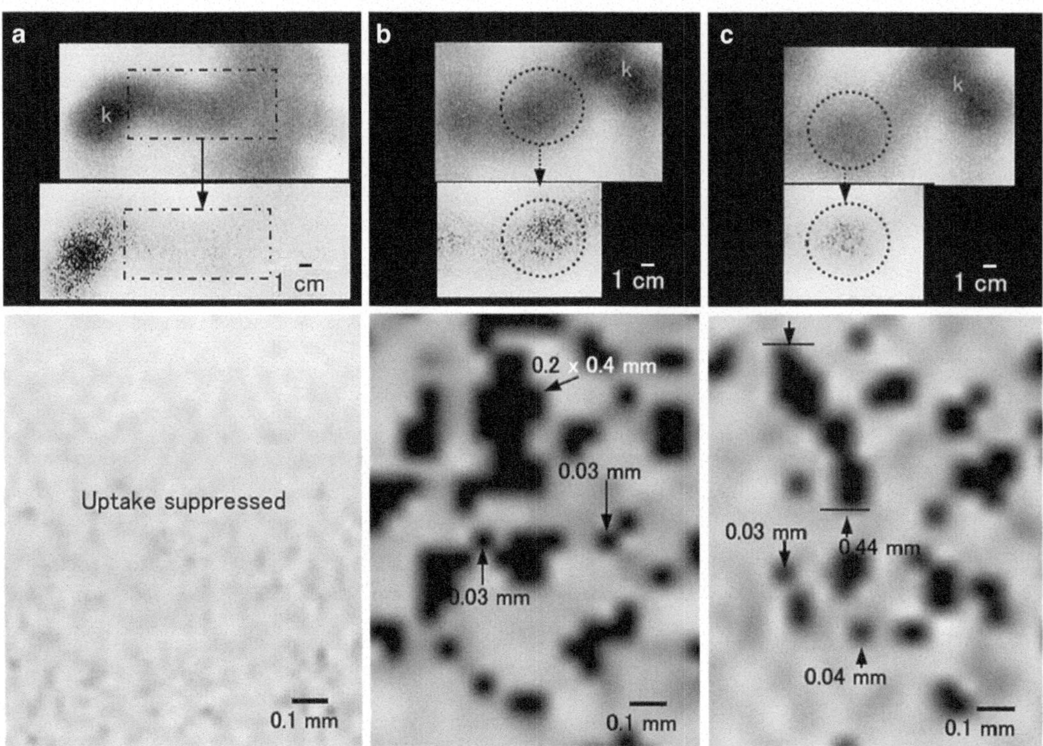

Fig. 4.5 Because unsuppressed individual pathological ^{99m}TC-HDP uptake in original GCPBS was too small to unaided eyes, 1-cm round region of interest in hypocenter was electronically 50-fold magnified to distinctly show micro tracer uptake for size assessment. The smallest one so measured was 30 μm in size. Top panel: (**a**) Normal control rat. (**b**) #1 rat post-contusion scan shows hypocenter (ring). (**c**) #2 rat post-contusion scan also shows hypocenter (ring). Bottom panel: (**a**) Normal control rat shows suppression of tracer uptake (frame). (**b**) #1 rat post-contusion scan shows a number of magnified microfractures in hypocenter (ring). (**c**) #2 rat post-contusion scan demonstrates similar microfreactures. The smallest callused microfracture measures 0.03 mm or 30 μm in size

malin. The fixed bone was bisected and decalcified using 10% formic acid for 7 days and then paraffin-embedded and sectioned at 7 μm. Sectioned slices were stained with hematoxylin and eosin. H&E stain and 50-fold magnified gamma correction pinhole scan were meticulously compared for histological validation (Fig. 4.6) and the correlative analysis confirmed excellent accord to exist between the results of gamma correction pinhole bone scan and H&E stain findings.

By separated correlation of the 50-fold magnified view of the trauma hypocenter in the rat's femoral shafts and high power (100×) H&E stain we were able to confirm and establish that there exists an excellent accord of the findings of enlarged gamma correction pinhole scan images and H&E stain (Fig. 4.7).

4.5 Findings of Conventional Radiograph, Seriated Naïve and Gamma Correction ^{99m}Tc-HDP Pinhole Bone Scans, and 50-Fold Magnified ^{99m}Tc-HDP Gamma Correction Callused Trabecular Microfracture for Size Measurement, and H&E Stain Validation

We systematically analyzed the findings of the conventional radiograph, seriated naïve, and gamma correction ^{99m}Tc-HDP pinhole bone scans, and 50-fold magnified ^{99m}Tc-HDP gamma correction of callused trabecular microfracture (CTMF). Technically, the size of individual TMF was measured in terms of a pixel using a magnifying lens and the results were histologically validated using H&E to systematically construct an objective, reasonable quantitation scale of CTMF.

4.5.1 Conventional Radiographic Findings of Callused Trabecular Microfracture in Young Rats

One normal control young rat in the first frame showed intact femur with actively growing physeal ossification centers in the knee and five injured rats showed falling iron-ball induced fractures in the femoral shaft (circle). Fractures in traumatized rats 3 and 5 were simple and the fractures in rats 1, 2, and 4 were compound with marked shaft deformity (Fig. 4.3).

4.5.2 Findings of Naïve ^{99m}Tc-HDP Pinhole Bone Scan and Gamma Correction Pinhole Bone Scan in Young Rats

One normal control young rat was presented in the first frame. It showed mild nominal physiological ^{99m}Tc-HDP uptake in the intact femoral shaft (*frame*) with intense tracer uptake occurring in physeal ossification centers in the knee. In contrast, the injured femoral shafts of five rats showed a focal area of increased tracer uptake in the hypocenter of falling iron-ball blow to the femoral shaft (*circle*). As mentioned above the tracer uptake was extremely small in size (Fig. 4.4) needing proper magnification for image and size assay as shown in Fig. 4.5.

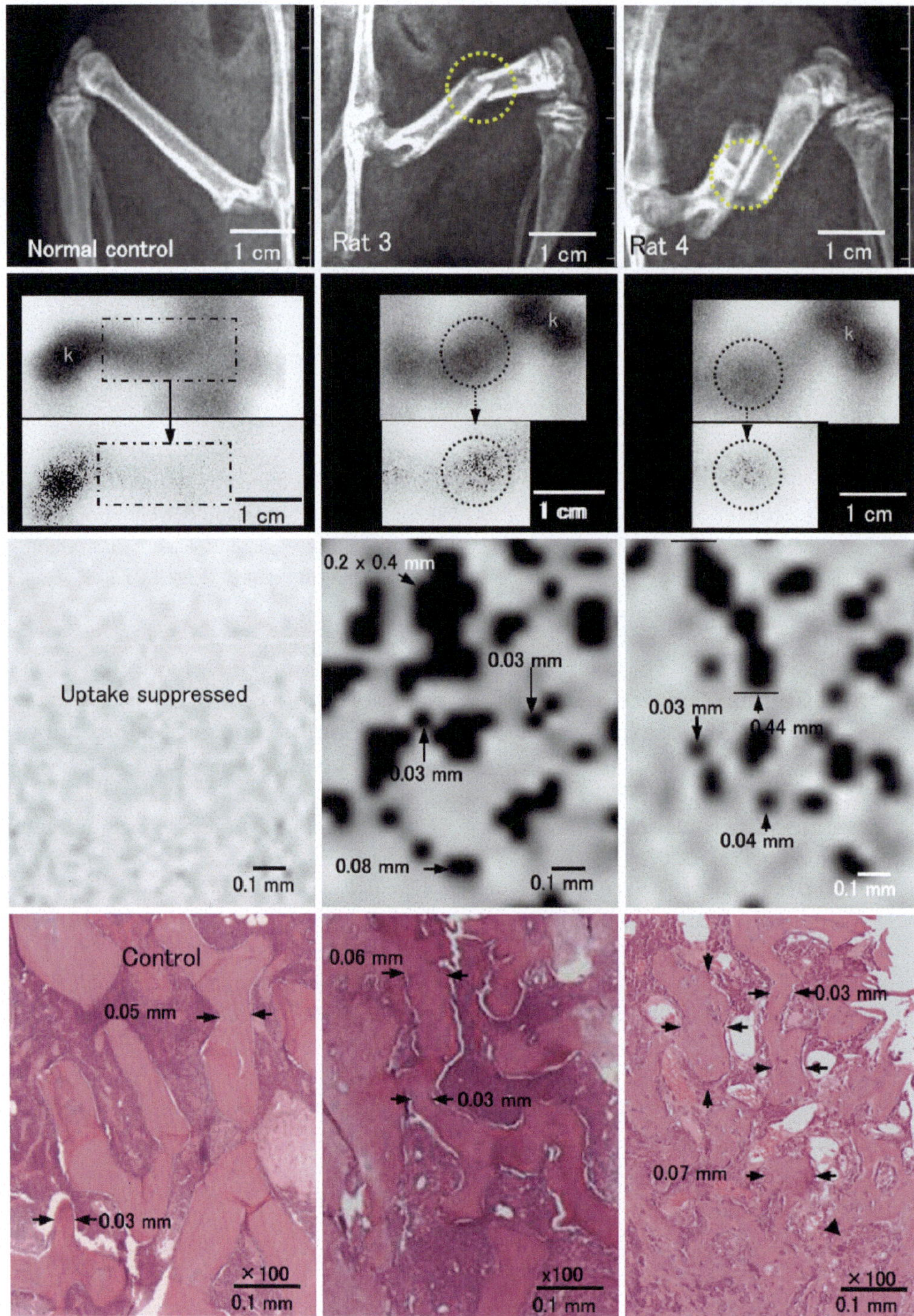

Fig. 4.6 Top panel: Radiographs of one normal control rat and two traumatized rats with different femoral shaft fracture induced by freely falling iron ball. Second panel: Naïve and ACDSee-7 gamma correction pinhole scans. The latter shows trabecular injuries. Third panel: 50 magnified views show callused trabecular microfractures. Bottom panel: H&E stain shows normal trabeculae and typical reactive endosteal rimming. The smallest measures 30 μm in size

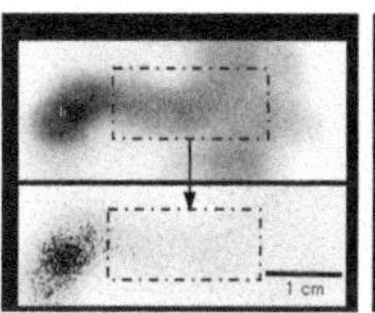
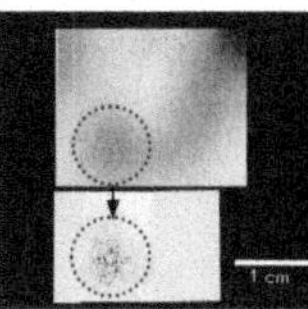
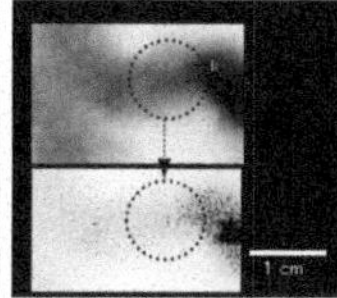
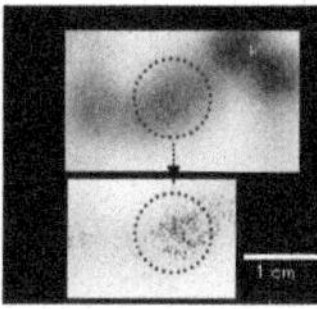
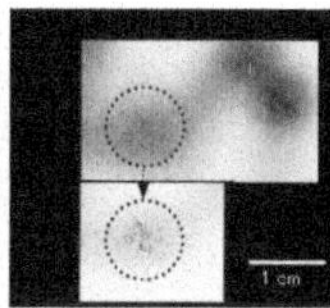
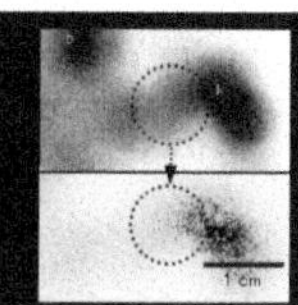

Fig. 4.7 One normal control young rat is presented in the first frame. It shows mild nominal physiological ^{99m}Tc-HDP uptake in the intact femoral shaft (frame) with intense tracer uptake in physeal ossification centers in the knee. In contrast, injured femoral shafts of five rats show focal area of increased tracer uptake in the hypocenter of falling iron-ball blow in the femoral shaft (circle). As shown in these cases actual pathological tracer uptake is extremely small in size needing appropriate magnification for image analysis and size assessment as will be seen in Fig. 4.8 (vide infra)

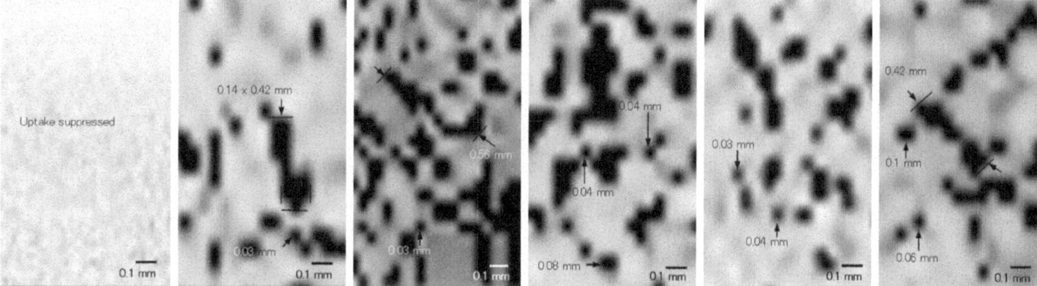

Fig. 4.8 One intact control young rat in the first frame shows neat suppression of mild ^{99m}Tc-HDP uptake in the intact femoral shaft and five traumatized rats show unsuppressed tracer uptake in variously shaped callused trabecular microfractures. Shapes are longitudinal, oblique, and transaxisal according to sectioning. The smallest one measures 0.03 mm or 30 μm in transaxial cut. Images were treated using ACDSee-7 gamma correction, which is handicapped by penumbra

4.5.3 Fifty-Fold Magnified ^{99m}Tc-HDP Gamma Correction View of Callused Trabecular Microfractures for Size Measurement

One intact control young rat in the first frame showed neat suppression of mild ^{99m}Tc-HDP uptake in the intact femoral shaft. However, all five traumatized rats showed unsuppressed high ^{99m}Tc-HDP uptake in variously shaped trabecular microfractures. The shapes are elongated, spotty, and slanted depending on the sectioning axis. The smallest one measured 30 μm in thickness when transaxially cut (Fig. 4.8).

4.5.4 Validation of ACDSee-7 Gamma Correction ^{99m}Tc-HDP Pinhole Bone Scan Findings of Trabecular Microfracture Using H&E Stain

We prospectively performed this reciprocal validation study on one normal control young rat and five injured rats by correlating the findings of ^{99m}Tc-HDP pinhole bone scan and H&E stain. The results first confirmed that the nominal tracer uptake in normal rat femoral shaft is neatly suppressed by gamma correction and second that there exists a high accord between the findings of gamma correction pinhole scan and H&E stain (Fig. 4.9). Gamma correction pinhole scan was 50-fold magnified so that it can be easily compared with H&E stain.

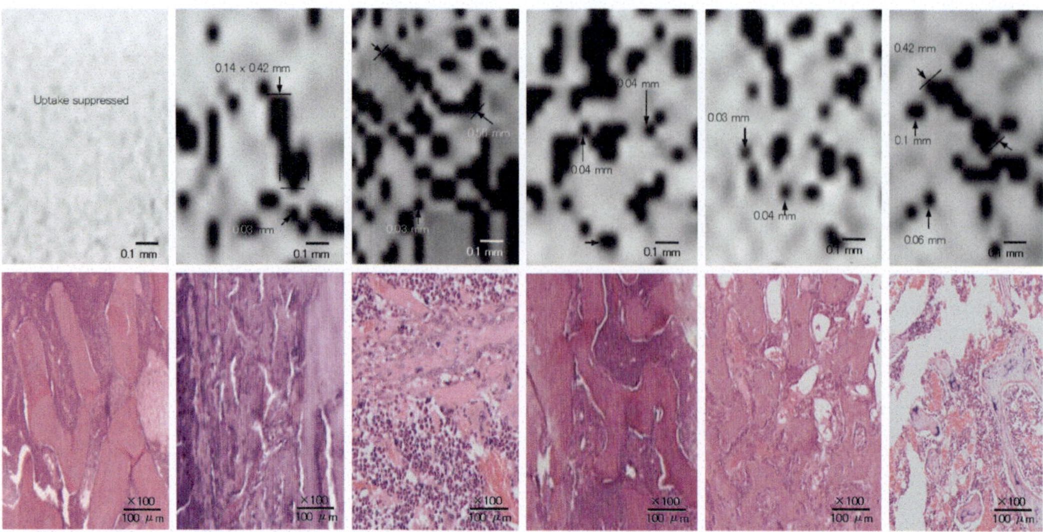

Fig. 4.9 This study presents the demonstration of ^{99m}Tc-HDP pinhole bone scan findings of one intact control rat to show neat suppression of nominal mild tracer uptake in intact femoral shaft. Then, gamma correction pinhole scan findings are histopathologically verified using H&E stain in all six rats including one control rat and five injured rats. Top panel: five traumatized rats show unsuppressed tracer uptake in variously shaped callused trabecular microfractures. They were cut longitudinally, obliquely, and transaxially. The smallest one measures 30 μm when transaxially cut. Bottom panel: H&E stain shows normal trabeculae in one control rat and variously shaped trabeculae with rimming and edema and/or hemorrhage in traumatized rats. Observe the blurry contour of injured trabeculae due to penumbra of ACDSee 7 gamma correction

References

Bahk YW, Jeon HS, Kim JM, et al. A novel use of gamma correction for precise ^{99m}Tc-HDP pinhole bone scan diagnosis and classification of knee occult fractures. Skeletal Radiol. 2010;39:807–81.

Bahk YW, Chung YA, Lee UY, Park SI. Gamma correction ^{99m}Tc-hydroxymethylene diphosphonate pinhole bone scan diagnosis and histopathological verification of trabecular contusion in young rats. Nucl Med Commun. 2016;37:988–91.

Bahk YW, Hwang SH, Lee UY, et al. Morphobiochemical diagnosis of acute trabecular microfractures using gamma correction Tc-99m HDP pinhole bone scan with histopathological verification. Medicine. 2017;96(45):e8419.

Bahk YW, Kim EE, Chung YA, et al. Precise differential diagnosis of acute bone marrow edema and hemorrhage and trabecular microfractures using naïve and gamma correction pinhole bone scans. J Int Med Res. 2019; https://doi.org/10.1177/0300060518819910.

Francis MD, Ferguson DL, Tofe AJ, et al. Comparative evaluation of three diphosphonates: in vitro adsorption (C-14 labeled) and in vivo osteogenic uptake (Tc-99m complexed). J Nucl Med. 1980;21:1185–9.

Gläser N, Kneubuehl BP, Zuber S, et al. Biomechanical examination of blunt trauma due to baseball bat blow to the head. J Forensic Biomech. 2011;2:F100601.

5 Preoperative Radiograph and Gamma Correction ^{99m}Tc-HDP Pinhole Scan of Femoral Neck Fracture in Patients

One day before surgery both conventional radiography and ^{99m}Tc-HDP pinhole bone scan were taken in order to anatomically and biochemically confirm the diagnosis of acute femoral neck fracture and thereby resulted in avascular necrosis of the femoral head in six consecutive patients (Bahk et al. 2017). Radiograph demonstrated fracture line (Fig. 5.1 top panel) and ^{99m}Tc-HDP pinhole bone scan showed obvious photon defect reflecting devascularized osteonecrosis, respectively (Fig. 5.1 bottom panel). Fractures were either scarcely recognized, slightly separated, or markedly deformed with fragment impaction and naïve pinhole scan straightforwardly showed typical photon defect in the devascularized femoral head (Fig. 5.1 bottom panel).

5.1 Conventional Radiography of Femoral Neck Fracture in Patients

Conventional radiograph was taken in each patient by a standardized radiographic machine. Radiographic exposure factors were 65–70 kVp, 35–40 mAs, and 100 cm source-image distance. AP radiograph showed the femoral neck fracture to vary in type. A simplified classification of fracture type was not clearly identified, well defined with mild fragment separation, or grossly contracted (Fig. 5.1 top panel).

5.2 ^{99m}Tc-HDP Pinhole Bone Scintigraphy of Femoral Neck Fracture

The incomparable diagnostic usefulness of ^{99m}Tc-HDP pinhole bone scan in the femoral neck fracture needs no emphasis because it can very uniquely provide the biochemical information in regards with the vascular state of fractured bone. For the convincing diagnosis of the devascularized state in the femoral head in the femoral neck fracture ^{99m}Tc-HDP pinhole bone scan was performed using a gamma camera system equipped with 4-mm pinhole collimator such as Siemens E-cam Signature gamma camera. Actually, the anterior pinhole scan of fractured hip joint was taken before surgery following the intravenous administration of 925–1110 MBq (25–30 mCi) ^{99m}Tc-HDP. The femoral head, removed by surgery for prosthesis, was then immediately subjected to pinhole bone scintigraphy to make a good use of the radioactivity remained undecayed from the 24-h preoperatively administered radionuclide (Bahk 2017). Each surgical specimen was confirmed to reserve a sufficient amount of radioactivity for

Y.-W. Bahk, *Imaging of Trabecular Microfracture and Bone Marrow Edema and Hemorrhage*,
https://doi.org/10.1007/978-981-15-4466-8_5

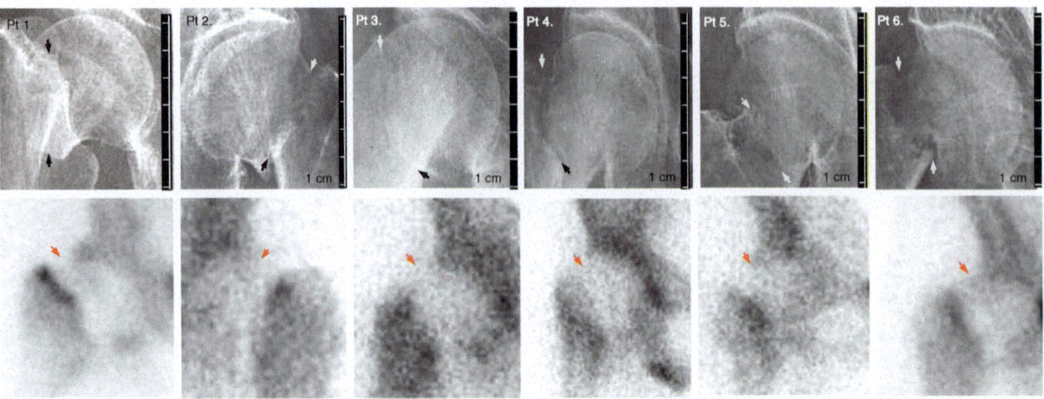

Fig. 5.1 Preoperative imaging diagnosis of femoral neck fracture in six patients. Top panel: preoperative anteroposterior radiographs show femoral neck fracture with osteoporosis (arrows). Fragments are either contracted, slightly separated, or straight. Bottom panel: preoperative ^{99m}Tc-HDP pinhole bone scan shows avascular photopenia in femoral heads (red arrows)

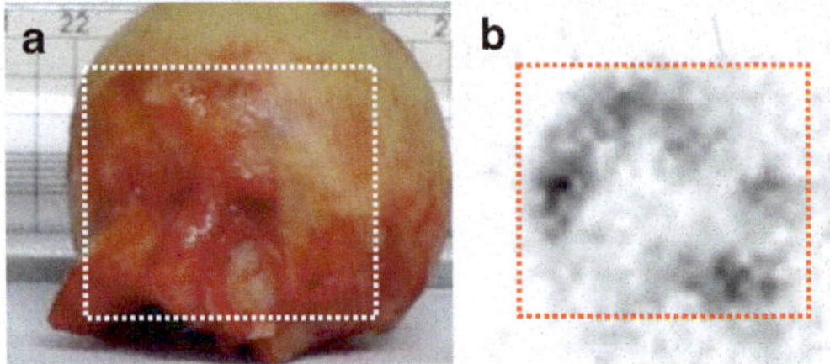

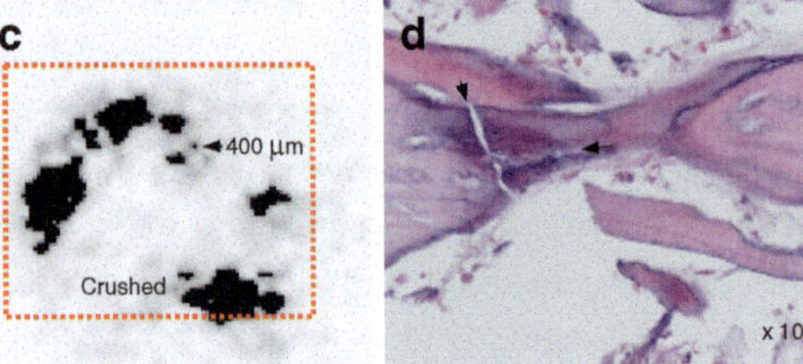

Fig. 5.2 Right femoral neck fracture in a 92-year-old-male. (**a**) Fresh surgical specimen shows femoral neck fracture and ROI in the femoral head (frame). (**b**) Naïve ^{99m}Tc-HDP pinhole scan shows areas of blurry tracer uptake with ROI (frame). (**c**) ACDSee-7 gamma correction pinhole scan shows crushed and 400-µm pinpointed microcalluses. (**d**) H&E stain shows lying down T-shaped fracture with base stained calcification (arrows)

useful bone scanning to attain naïve and gamma correction scan profiles. In the meantime, the 10%-formalin solution cleansed cut surface of surgical specimen was scrutinized by surface microscope to record and confirm the presence of actively forming CTMF (callused trabecular microfractures (Fig. 5.2a). The specimen was then examined using ^{99m}Tc-HDP pinhole scanning to attain the naïve pinhole scan image that showed nonspecific blurry uptake in injured bone (Fig. 5.2b) and subsequent gamma correction (Fig. 5.2c) highlighted CTMF with unsuppressed tracer uptake. The smallest CTMF in this cased was 400 µm and H&E stain confirmed linear microfractures with classic base stain (Fig. 5.2d). Furthermore, the devascularized femoral head in the femoral neck fracture can be imaged most distinctly by this simple method (Fig. 5.3b).

5.3 Advantages of Gamma Correction ^{99m}Tc-HDP Pinhole Bone Scan in Diagnosis of Trabecular Microfractures and Other Diseases of Irregular Bones

In the human body, there are a number of large and small irregular bones with various diseases including trauma, inflammation, infection, tumor, and others. For the precise diagnosis of those diseases in irregular bones gamma correction ^{99m}Tc-HDP pinhole bone scan is considered to play an important and more often than not irreplaceable role, which is highly effective yet economical (Bahk 2017). Following cases are presented as typical examples of such diseases. They are the atlas and axis (C1 and C2) of the cervical spine at

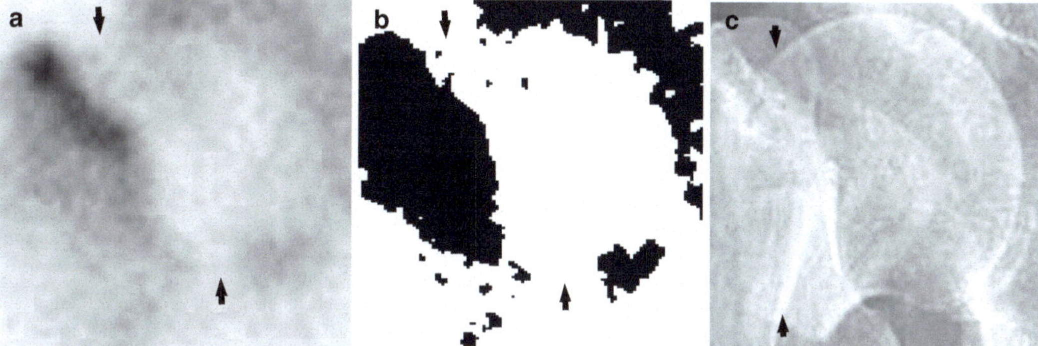

Fig. 5.3 The most definitive imaging demonstration of avascular necrosis using ACDSee-10 gamma correction of the right femoral head due to femoral neck fracture in a 72-year-old male. (**a**) Naïve anterior ^{99m}Tc-HDP pinhole scan shows decreased tracer uptake in the femoral head (arrows). Mild tracer uptake is seen in vascularized acetabulum and the intertrochanteric zone. (**b**) Impressively, gamma correction pinhole scan shows large bright photopenia in devascularized femoral head. In contrast, the vascularized bones are presented as blackened areas. (**c**) Anteroposterior radiograph shows irregular femoral neck fracture with contracted bone fragments (arrows)

the skull base, thin flat nasal bones, small articular U-shaped hyoid bone in the anterior neck, the irregular triangular scapula, the dimpled-protruded articular elbow bones, complex wrist bones, the pelvis with basin-flat iliac bones and joints and back walling sacrum, and compound ankle. Actually, the gamma correction pinhole scan is able to efficiently and rather uniquely diagnose trabecular bone pathologies in those bones. Following cases are typical examples of highly advantageous use of gamma correction ^{99m}Tc-HDP pinhole bone scan.

Case 1

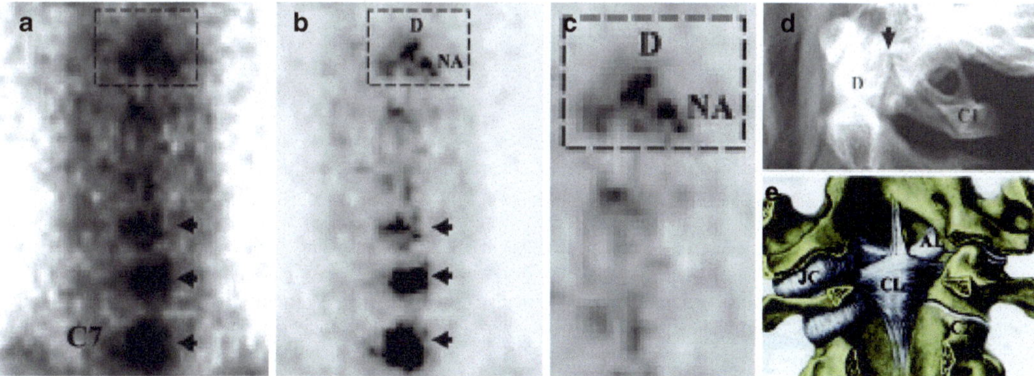

Being located at the skull base C1 and C2 vertebrae are anatomically complex and clinically perilous bones to manipulate, especially when they are traumatized. Case 1 figure demonstrates neck sprain with a small fracture of the odontoid process along with obvious C5-7 spinous process fractures. (**a**) Naïve ^{99m}Tc-HDP pinhole scan of the cervical spine shows nonspecific blurry tracer uptake in the atlantoaxial complex (frame) and obvious button-like uptake in the C5-7 spinous processes. (**b**) Gamma correction view individually demonstrates small spotty tracer uptake in the dens (D) and C1 neural arch (NA) as well as C5-7 spinous processes (arrows). (**c**) Twofold magnified view of the dens convincingly visualizes pathological tracer uptake in the dens and C1 neural arch (NA). (**d**) Lateral conventional radiograph shows subtle fractures of the atlantoaxial joint and dens (arrow). (**e**) Topography shows normal anatomical detail of C1 and 2 (Adopted from "Anatomy". Clements CD. 2nd ed. Urban & Schwarzenberg, München 1981)

Case 2

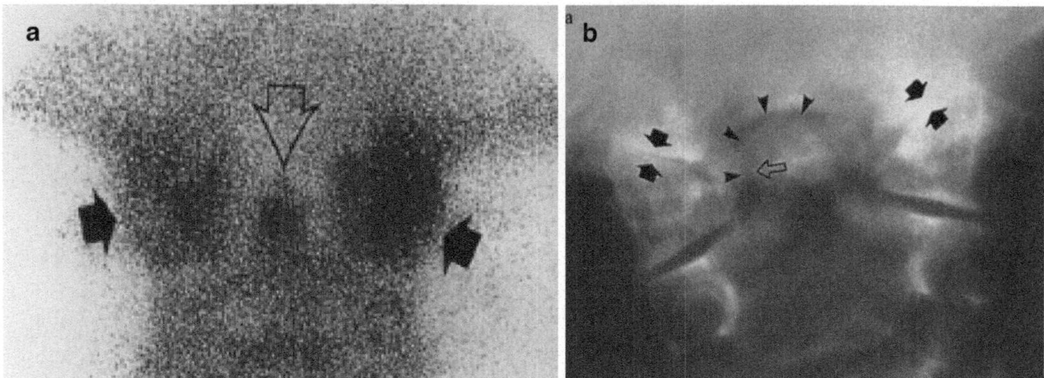

Anatomico-radiobiochemical diagnosis of rheumatoid arthritis of the uppermost cervical spine in a 70-year-old female diagnosed using gamma correction ^{99m}Tc-HDP pinhole bone scan. (**a**) Posterior pinhole scan shows moderately increased tracer uptake in the right occipitoatlantal joint and markedly increased tracer uptake in the left occipitoatlantal joint (frame). The odontoid process is also affected showing increased tracer uptake (large open arrow). (**b**) Anteroposterior radiograph shows the narrowing and blurring of the superior articular facets of the atlas (apposing arrows) and atlantoaxial joint (arrowheads)

Case 3

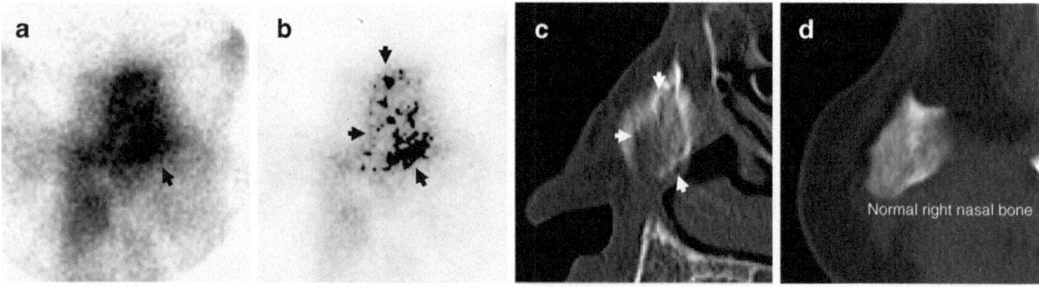

Characteristic speckled and pinpointed microfractures of the left nasal bone in a 68-year-old female diagnosed using gamma correction ^{99m}Tc-HDP pinhole bone scan. (**a**) Anterior ^{99m}Tc-HDP pinhole scan shows nonspecific blurry tracer uptake in the left nasal bone (arrow). The nasal bone is intact. (**b**) ACDSee-7 gamma correction scan (gamma = 80) highlights a number of small irregular mottled and spotty tracer uptake of microfractures with penumbra (arrows). (**c**) Sagittal MDCT of the injured left nasal bone shows several small dark spots of fractures intermixed with a fine linear shadow of the anterior ethmoidal nerve groove. (**d**) The right nasal bone is intact. Observe high sensitivity and unique diagnostic specificity of gamma correction pinhole bone scan in this case. Unsuppressed positive ^{99m}Tc-HDP uptake denotes fractured bone with active osteoneogenesis. Radiograph is unable to differentiate microfractures from vascular and innervation channels

Case 4

Accidentally highlighted ^{99m}Tc-HDP uptake is shown in a chronic tender fracture of the intercornual joint of the hyoid bone in a 33-year-old male dental patient. (**a**) Naïve pinhole scan shows a small blurry tracer uptake with high tracer uptake in the central core of the right intercornual joint which is ankylosed (arrow). (**b**) ACDSee-10 gamma correction view shows neatly highlighted microfractures (arrow). There are three archipelagic and multiple pin-point microfractures in the left mandibular molar teeth due to alveolitis. (**c**) Radiograph shows the ankylosis of the intercornual joint of the hyoid bone (arrow)

Case 5

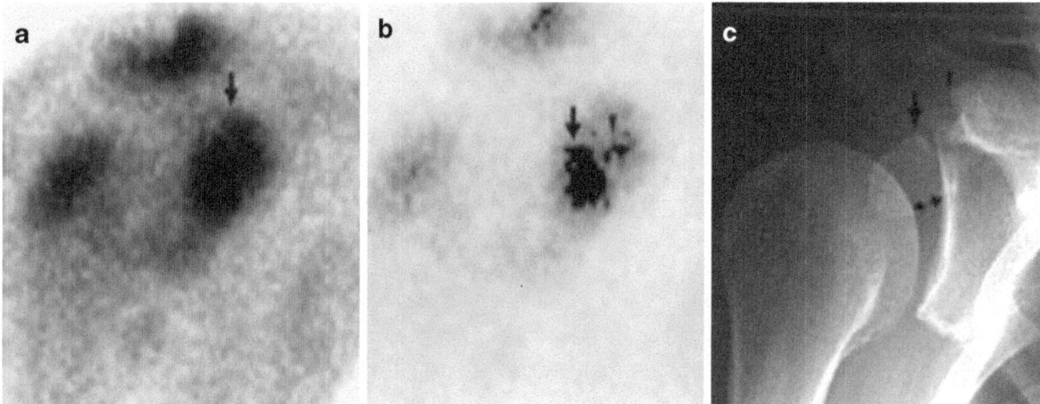

Ovoid tracer uptake is seen in a dislocated fracture fragment of the corcoid process of the right scapula in a 58-year-old male. (**a**) Naïve anterior ^{99m}Tc-HDP pinhole bone scan of the right shoulder girdle shows intense blurry tracer uptake in the coracoid process region. (**b**) ACDSee-7 gamma correction view shows the suppression of blurry tracer uptake highlighting unsuppressed tracer uptake in the coracoid bone tip which is fractured and separated from the scapular body but with preserved blood flow. The shaggy tip of the broken process also shows stippled tracer uptake (arrowhead). (**c**) Radiograph shows the separation of fragment (arrow) and joint subluxation (paired arrowheads)

Case 6

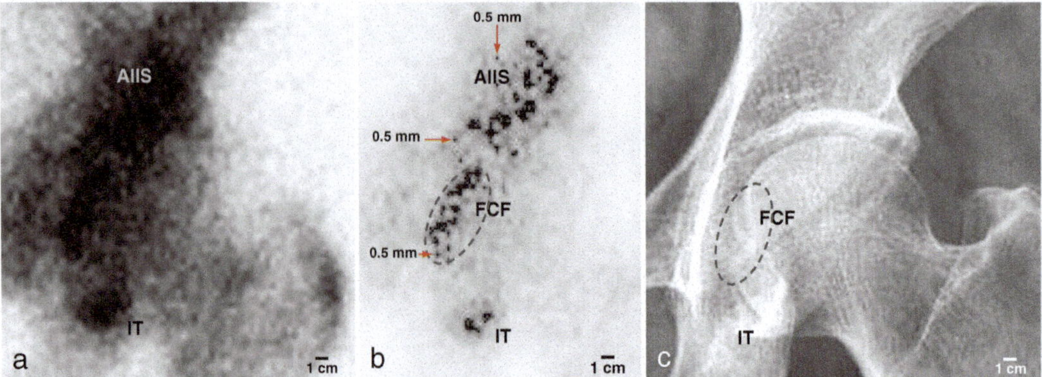

Microfractures occurred in the left hip joint bones in a 56-year-old female due to motor vehicle accident. (**a**) Anterior ^{99m}Tc-HDP pinhole bone scan of the left hip joint shows bizarre nonspecific blurry tracer uptake in the hip joint bones including the anteroinferior iliac spine (AIIS). (**b**) Gamma correction view shows multiple pinpointed and mottled areas of unsuppressed tracer uptake in the anterior inferior iliac spine region (AIIS), acetabular roof, fovea capitis femoris (FCF), and ischial tuberosity (IT). (**c**) Anteroposterior radiograph shows irregular roughened bones in the fovea capitis femoris (FCF) and ischial tuberosity (IT)

Case 7

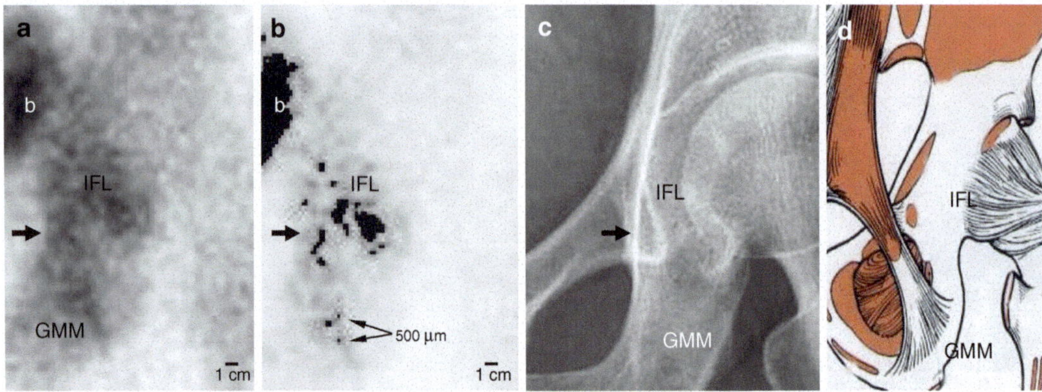

Rare immobilization pressure enthesitis occurred at the insertions of the right ischiofemoral ligament (IFL) and gluteus maximus muscle (GMM) in a 61-year-old female. This post-craniectomy enthesitis resulted from 4-day-long immobilization on a patient bed. (**a**) ^{99m}TC-HDP pinhole scan shows nonspecific blurry tracer uptake. *b* is urinary bladder. (**b**) Gamma correction view shows multiple trabecular fractures with unsuppressed tracer uptake. The smallest uptake measures 500 μm in size. (**c**) Radiograph shows regional anatomy including the ischiofemoral ligament (IFL) and the gluteus maximus muscle (GMM). (**d**) Topography of stressed ligament and muscle insertions. Anatomy, 2nd ed. 1981. Permission obtained from Clements CD. München: Urban & Schwarzenberg

Case 8

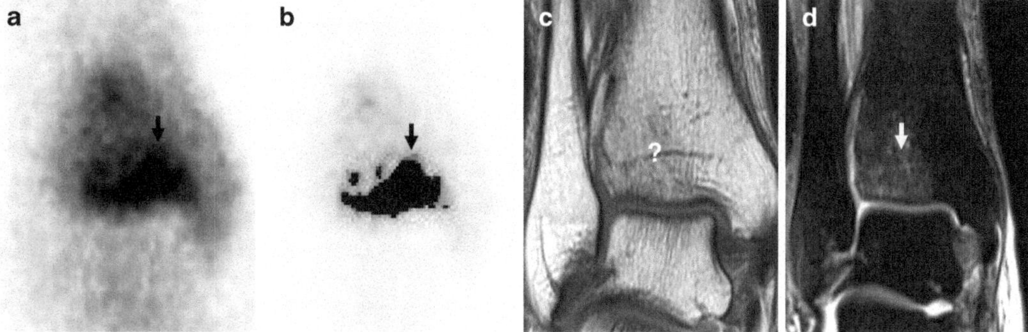

Gamma correction pinhole scan shows distinct fractures in the distal end of the right tibia where the torn joint capsule is tightly attached. The patient is a 63-year-old male. (**a**) Naive ^{99m}Tc-HDP pinhole bone scan shows nonspecific blurry high tracer uptake in the distal tibial end. It consists of higher and lower uptake denoting fracture and edema, respectively. (**b**) ACDSee-7 gamma correction highlights the high uptake of fracture with the low tracer uptake in edema suppressed (arrow). (**c**) T1-weighted FS MRI (480/10) shows only suspicious signal intensity change (?). (**d**) T2-weighted MRI (2800/31) shows bright signal intensity which is not distinct as bone scan uptake (arrow). Observe obvious differences in the diagnostic efficacy of bone scan and MRI in this case. Such a difference is not rare between 3D and 2D images

Case 9

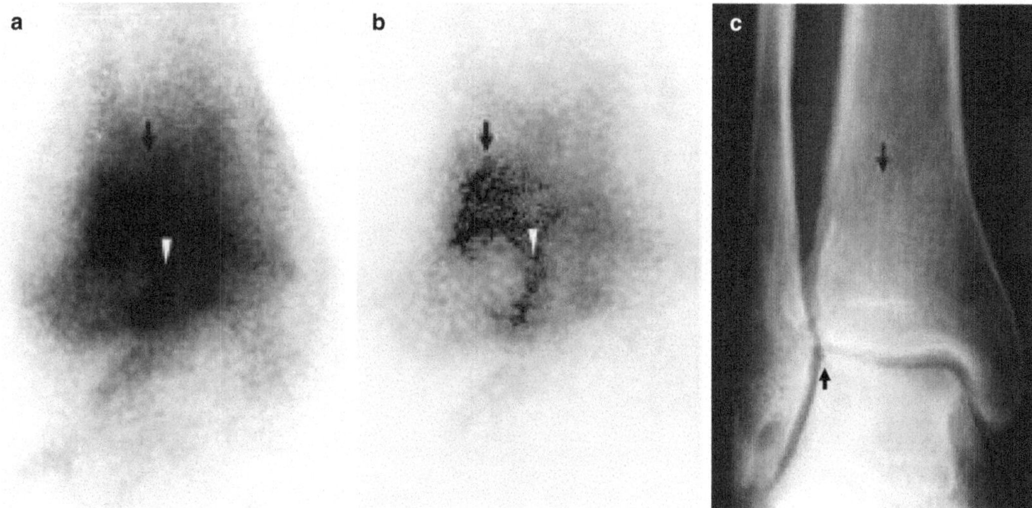

Gamma correction ^{99m}Tc-HDP pinhole bone scan shows blurry high ^{99m}Tc-HDP uptake in Brodie's abscess in the distal end of the right tibial shaft which penetrated down into the talus (arrowhead) in a 54-year-old male. (**a**) Naïve anterior pinhole bone scan shows blurry tracer uptake in the distal tibial diaphysis with an inferior extension (arrowhead). (**b**) Gamma correction view clearly demonstrates a small inferior penetration of infection into the talus across joint. (**c**) Conventional radiograph shows mild osteosclerosis (top arrow) with joint space narrowing (bottom arrow). Observe the incomparable advantage of gamma correction pinhole bone scanning

This case presentation is meant to confirm the uniqueness and usefulness of gamma correction pinhole scan as a fundamental imaging diagnostic tool of small irregular anatomical structures. In particular, the anatomical diagnosis by this method is specifically endorsed by bone metabolic profile in terms of osteoneogenesis.

References

Bahk YW. Combined scintigraphic and radiographic diagnosis of bone and joint diseases with gamma correction interpretation. 5th ed. Heidelberg/Berlin: Springer; 2017.

Bahk YW, Hwang SH, Lee UY, et al. Morphobiochemical diagnosis of acute trabecular microfractures using gamma correction Tc-99m HDP pinhole bone scan with histopathological verification. Medicine. 2017;96(45):e8419.

Gamma Correction ^{99m}Tc-HDP Pinhole Bone Scan Demonstration of Callused Trabecular Microfracture

6

Gamma correction ^{99m}Tc-HDP pinhole bone scan can uniquely demonstrate CTMF along with bone metabolic profile. The smallest CTMF imaged on gamma correction pinhole bone scan measures 200 μm in size and this size is equivalent to one pixel. We carried out a seriated naïve and gamma correction pinhole bone scan study with histological verification to fundamentally establish a morphobiochemical diagnostic basis of CTMF in six surgical specimens of femoral neck fracture. Specimens were attained from femoral neck fracture surgery performed for prosthetic replacement. After cleansing with 10% formalin solution the broken surface of the specimen was scrutinized using a surgical surface microscope to confirm that seed-pearly callused microcalluses were formed (Fig. 6.1). As the extension of the study, the surgical specimens were further imaged using ^{99m}Tc-HDP pinhole bone scan and then serially treated by gamma correction, earlier using ACDSee-7 version and lately using ACDSee 10 version. The former version treated image showed penumbra, but the latter version image showed no penumbra (vide infra).

The anatomical changes of injured trabeculae shown on naïve and gamma correction pinhole bone scans, surface microphotograph, and H&E stain were meticulously correlated for histological validation. In addition, the suppressed ^{99m}Tc-HDP uptake in edema and hemorrhage and the unsuppressed uptake in CTMF were assessed by ACDSee-10 gamma correction and the results confirmed that GCPBS characteristically suppressed edema and hemorrhage uptake to neatly highlight CTMF. The shapes of highlighted CTMF were pinpointed, speckled, round, ovoid, rod-like, geographic and crushed, and sizes could be measured using the pixelized method (Jung et al. 2016) or magnifying optic lens method and the smallest CTMF was 0.23 mm in size as measured by the former method and 200 μm by the latter method. On the other hand, GCPBS was able to biochemically discern the callused microfracture with enhanced ^{99m}Tc-HDP uptake. Consequently, the microfracture with unsuppressed tracer uptake could be distinguished from the uncalcified tissues with suppressed tracer uptake. Thus, gamma correction ^{99m}Tc-HDP pinhole bone scan is proven to be highly useful for the specific diagnosis of CTMF (Fig. 6.1 top panel).

Trabecular microfracture ubiquitously occurs in osteoporosis (Vernon-Roberts and Pirie 1973), contusion (Mandalia and Henson 2008), aseptic osteonecrosis (McFarland and Frost 1961), inflammatory, metabolic, and bone tumors (Bahk 2013), and even in physiological activity and daily works (Fazzarali 1993). Clinically, trabecular microfracture is negligible when localized, but when widespread or systemic it may well become a condition to disturb the equilibrium

Y.-W. Bahk, *Imaging of Trabecular Microfracture and Bone Marrow Edema and Hemorrhage*,
https://doi.org/10.1007/978-981-15-4466-8_6

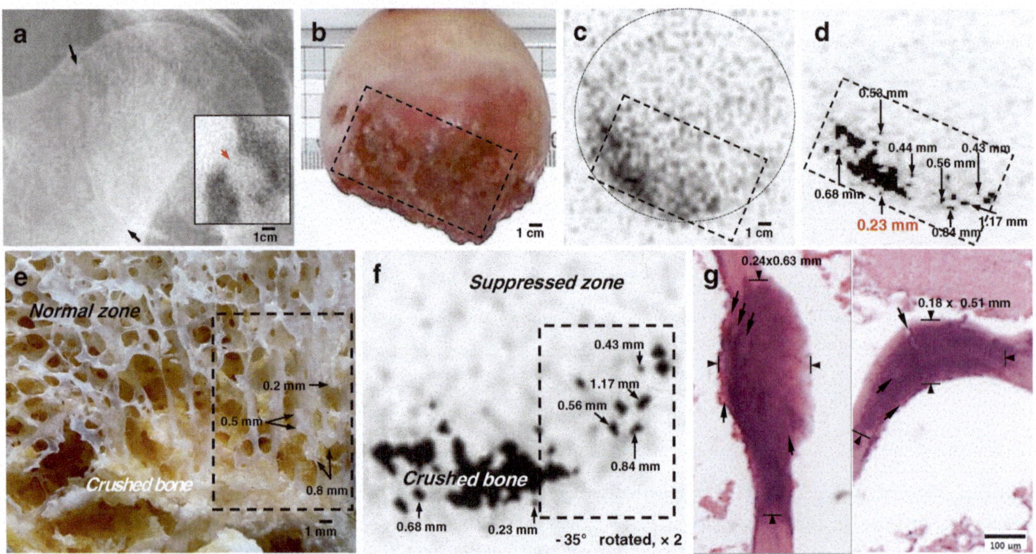

Fig. 6.1 ACDSee-7 gamma correction pinhole bone scan shows callused trabecular microfractures with remniscent penumbra. (**a**) Radiograph shows fracture (*arrows*) and inset pinhole bone scan shows photon defect. (**b**) Fresh surgical specimen shows fracture surface roughened by seed-pearly callused microfractures (*frame*). (**c**) Naïve ^{99m}Tc-HDP pinhole scan shows nonspecific blurry tracer uptake (*frame*). (**d**) Gamma correction view shows suppression of blurry tracer uptake rendering microfractures highlighted. The smallest one measures 0.23 mm or 230 µm in size. (**e**) Surgical surface microscope shows trabecular microfractures (*frame*) with the smallest one measuring 0.2 mm in size. (**f**) 35°counterclockwise rotated and ×2 magnified view of gamma correction pinhole scan to match with (**e**). (**g**) H&E stain shows typical base stain (*arrows*)

state of the whole skeletal system manifesting as a major debilitating disease, especially in the aged population (Tassani 2014). It heals by callus formation, an aggregation of woven bone, presenting in forms of nodular, fusiformed, angulated, or arched-bridge-like trabecular lesion (Fazzarali 1993). Histologically, H&E stain reveals linear fracture to be either complete, incomplete, or poorly defined (Fig. 6.2 top panel) and gamma correction pinhole scan shows the unsuppressed tracer uptake to be archipelagic, dotted, and pinpointed in shape (Fig. 6.2 bottom panel).

We consider that such gamma correction ^{99m}Tc-HDP pinhole scan imaging of CTMF may be clinically used as a convenient validation ground instead of H&E stain when clinical situation needs. It is to be known that gamma correction pinhole scans, both ACDSee 7 and ACDSee 10 versions, can highlight CTMF but ACDSee 7 is handicapped by penumbra, which annoyingly blurs trabecular definition (Fig. 6.3). Indeed, when processed using ACDSee 7 gamma correction there may remain penumbra but it can be neatly avoided using upgraded ACDSee 10 version (Fig. 6.3). Moreover, the imaging sensitivity of ACDSee 10 is significantly enhanced to neatly demonstrate even smaller trabecular microfracture, which measures 200 µm in size.

Historically, trabecular microfractures began to draw researcher's attention in the early 1960s as they were first observed in the necrotized femoral head in patients with hypercortisolism (McFarland and Frost 1961). In the beginning, conventional radiography was used for their study and decades later MRI followed it. The usefulness of MRI for the diagnosis of TMF was first published by Yao and Lee (1988). They noted high signal intensity in T2-weighted image and speckled or linear low signal intensity in the T1-weighted image in contused knee bones. Their results were years later confirmed in a larger number of patients (Mink and Deutch 1989). In the meantime, Rangger et al. (1998) performed a histopathological study on cancellous bone microfractures newly using cryosec-

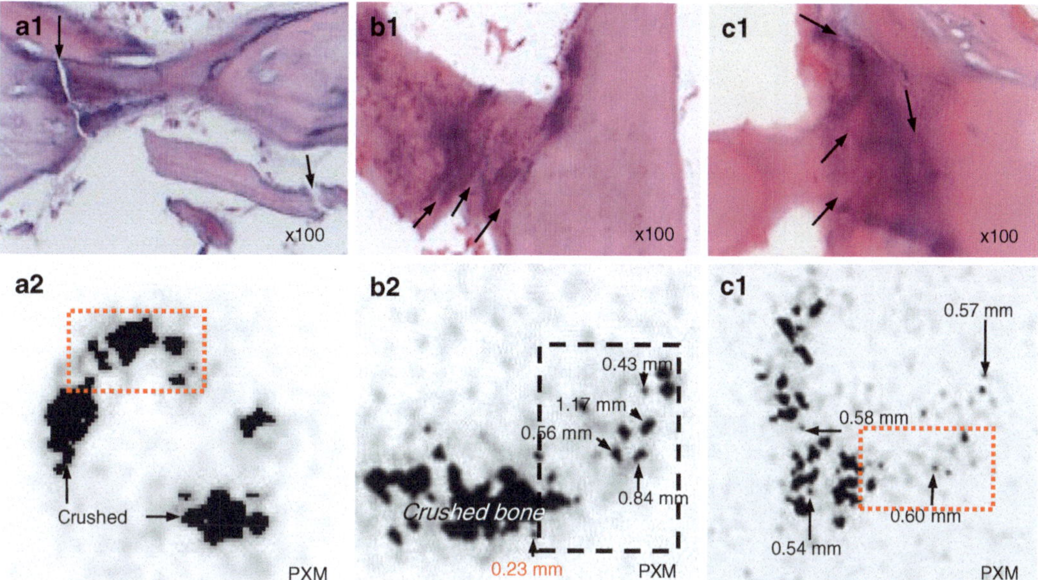

Fig. 6.2 Trabecular microfractures can be either sharply defined (**a1**), intermediary defined (**b1**), or blurry defined (**c1**) in type. The size of microcallus was measured by pixelized measurement (PXM) of the Monte Carlo simulation study (Yoon et al. 2014). The smallest callus was 0.23 mm or 230 μm as shown in b2 (red). Tomographic image of prompt gamma-ray emission from boron neutron capture therapy: a Monte Carlo simulation study. Appl Phys Lett 2014;104:083521

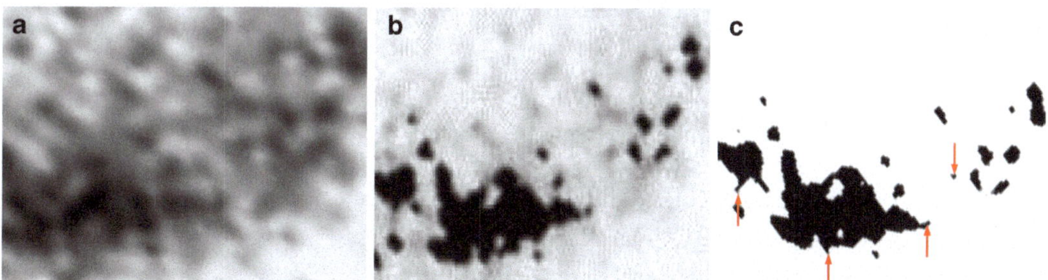

Fig. 6.3 Neat definition and higher sensitivity of ACDSee-10 gamma correction image compared to conventional ACDSee-7 gamma correction in a 72-year-old female patient. (**a**) Naïve ^{99m}Tc-HDP pinhole scan shows nonspecific blurry tracer uptake. (**b**) ACDSee-7 gamma correction pinhole scan shows callused trabecular microfractures and archipelagic fractures with unsuppressed blurry contour due to penumbra. (**c**) ACDSee-10 gamma correction view shows neatly sharpened microfracture contour (red arrows). Smaller calluses are additively shown due to increased image sensitivity

tion and their work was followed by an MRI investigation of bone contusion using a swine model (Ryu et al. 2000). In the meantime, micro-computed tomography (micro-CT) was developed (Klinstroem et al. 2014) and micro magnetic resonance imaging by Song and Wehrli (1999). And most recently we found that ^{99m}Tc-HDP pinhole bone scan can handily image CTMF when treated by gamma correction in young rat (Bahk et al. 2016) (Figs. 6.4 and 6.5) and also in the surgical specimen of femoral neck fracture in patient (Bahk et al. 2017) (Fig. 6.6).

Actually, GCPBS could reliably differentiate CTMF from normal trabeculae as the ^{99m}Tc-HDP uptake in the former is markedly enhanced using gamma correction, whereas the mild

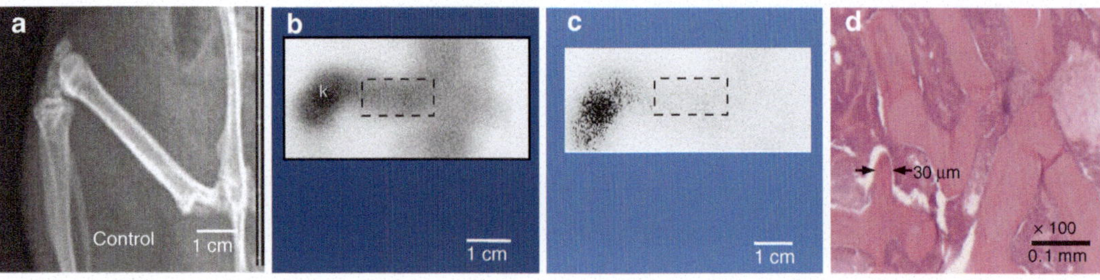

Fig. 6.4 Normal control young rat. (**a**) Radiograph of a normal control rat. (**b**) Animal pinhole scan shows an intact femur with physiological tracer uptake in the growing knee bones (*k*) and femoral shaft (frame). (**c**) Gamma correction view shows neat suppression of tracer uptake. (**d**) H&E stain shows scarcely visible intact endosteum

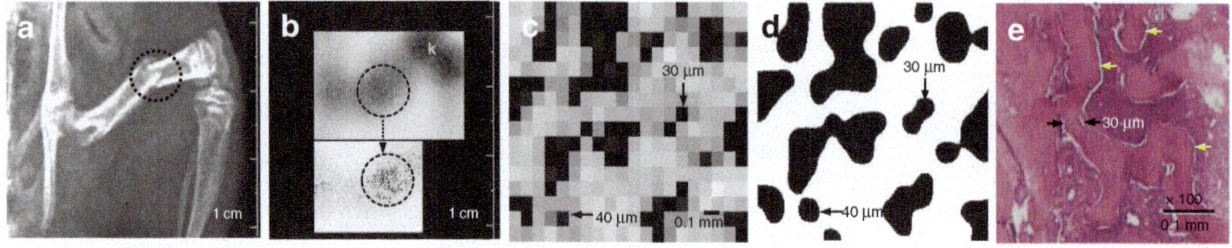

Fig. 6.5 Mid-femoral shaft fracture and contusion created by falling iron-ball method in a young rat. (**a**) Radiograph shows angular fracture with occult contusion (*circle*). (**b**) Top frame is ^{99m}Tc-HDP animal pinhole scan showing increased tracer uptake in the hypocenter (circle) and bottom frame is gamma correction pinhole scan showing highlighted pinpoint tracer uptake (*circle*). k is growing plate in the knee. (**c**) ×200 ACDSee-7 gamma correction view shows magnified callused microtrabecular tracer uptake with blurry penumbral contour (*arrow*). (**d**) ACDSee-10 gamma correction view shows neatly defined callused trabecular microfractrure. (**e**) H&E stain shows well defined reactive endosteal rimming (*yellow arrows*)

uptake in normal and moderate uptake in edema and hemorrhage is cleanly suppressed (Bahk 2013; Bahk et al. 2010). Our histological studies in young rats and surgical specimens proved that morphobiochemical diagnosis of calcifying CTMF is possible. In this connection Francis et al. published in 1980 an important experimental study that showed higher ^{99m}Tc-diphosphonates uptake occur in osteoneogenesis in acutely healing fractures in Sprague-Dawley rats. They found ^{99m}Tc-diphosphonates to be more richly adsorbed onto amorphous calcium phosphate which has more osteogenetic sites than the crystalline hydroxyapatite of intact bone. We similarly performed a histobiochemical study using rats to afresh confirm that the morpho-radiobiochemical diagnosis of actively calcifying CTMF is possible using GCPBS (Fig. 6.5). We continuously and additionally performed a clinical study using surgical specimens of devascularized femoral heads removed for the treatment of femoral neck fracture as recruited from six patients. All patients individually agreed to and signed an informed consent for this study, which was approved by the Institutional review board. The age of patients ranged from 72 to 92 years (mean = 78.4) and genders were 3 males and 3 females. The fracture involved the right femoral neck in five patients and the left femoral neck in one patient. The femoral head was surgically removed 3–7 days after fracture for prosthesis (Fig. 6.6). For information, this study was published under the title of "Morphobiochemical diagnosis of acute trabecular microfractures using gamma correction Tc-99mm HDP pinhole bone scan with histopathological verification" (Bahk et al. 2017).

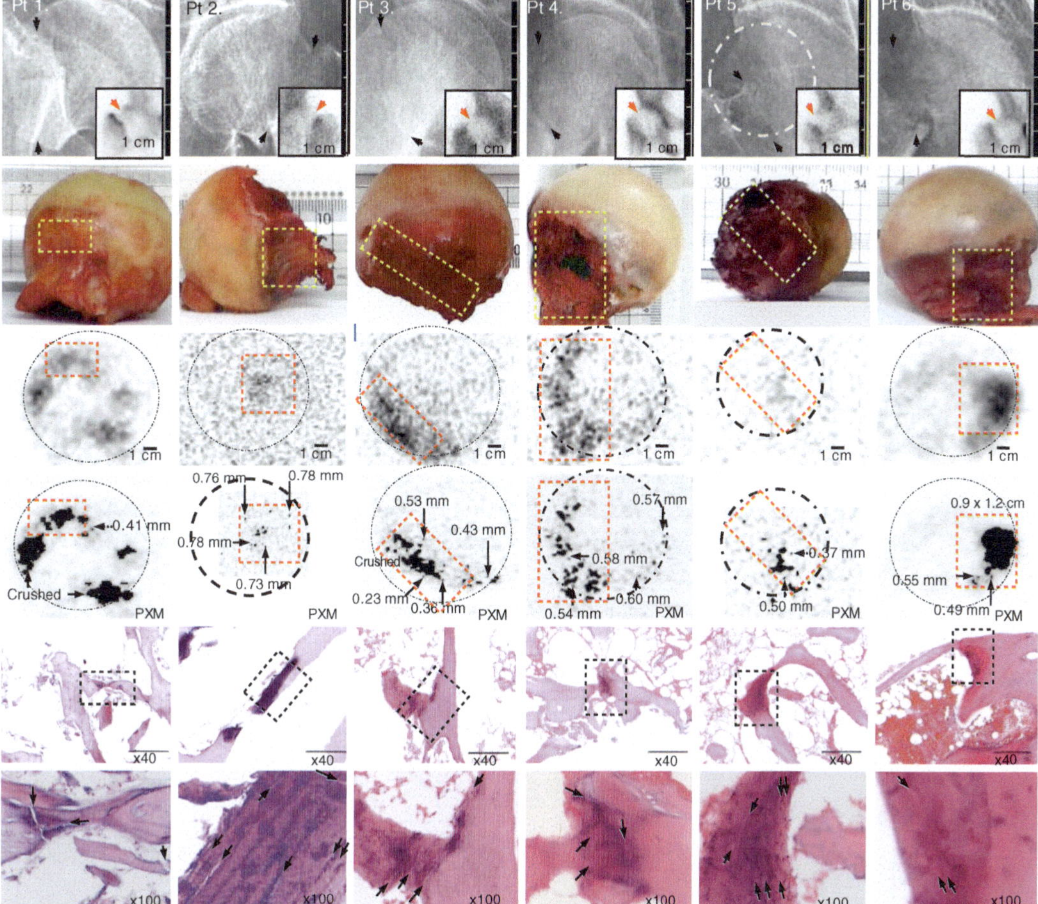

Fig. 6.6 Patients, examinations, and results of ACDSee-7 gamma correction. Top panel: preoperative radiographs show femoral neck fracture with osteoporosis (arrowhead). Inset is preoperative bone scan showing avascular photopenia in femoral heads (red arrows). Second panel: fresh surgically removed femoral heads show neck fracture with a ruler for basic size measurement and selection of region of interest (frame). Third panel: the naive pinhole scans of specimen show blurry pathological and background ^{99m}Tc-HDP uptake (frame). Fourth panel: post GCPBS show unwashed high tracer uptake in pinpoint, speckled, rod-like, geographic, and crushed fractures. Size was measured by the pixelized method (PXM). Note that the tracer uptake in normal and edema and/or hemorrhage is washed out. Fifth panel: low power view (×40) H&E stain shows scanty trabecular microfractures with callus formation in porotic bone replaced by fat cells. Patient 6 shows hemorrhage. Bottom panel: High power view of H&E stain (×100) shows linear microfractures in all patients. Fractures are well defined in Patients 1–3 and poorly defined in Patients 4–6 (black arrows). The definition of fracture appeared unrelated with days of fracture

6.1 Histological Validation of Gamma Correction ^{99m}Tc-HDP Pinhole Bone Scan Findings

Necrotized femoral head due to femoral neck fracture was surgically removed for arthroplasty 24 h after the diagnostic confirmation of the osteonecrosis using both radiography (Fig. 6.6 top panel) and vascular bone necrosis using ^{99m}Tc-HDP pinhole bone scanning (Fig. 6.6 top panel inset) in six consecutive patients. Regular imaging study performed was naïve ^{99m}Tc-HDP pinhole scanning and its gamma correction to specifically demonstrate trabecular microfracture observed by surgical microscopy in each patient (Fig. 6.6 second panel). Individual fracture was further assessed on pinhole bone scan that was serially processed using gamma correction (Fig. 6.6 third and fourth panels). Finally thereafter, CTMF shown on GCPBS and H&E stain were meticulously intercorrelated for histological verification (Fig. 6.6 fifth and sixth panels). As anticipated, GCPBS showed large archipelagic and small variously shaped trabecular microfractures with intense unsuppressed tracer uptake (Fig. 6.7b). As explained, the radioactivity so detected was derived from the un-decayed residua of the ^{99m}Tc-HDP intravenously administered to each patient 24-hr before surgery. The amount of tracer, aperture-to-object distance, field of view size, and matrix size were 1.0–1.07 GBq (3.7–4.0 mCi), 12 cm, 14 × 14 cm, and 256 × 256, respectively. Those data were needed for mathematic calculation of pixelized measurement although this complicated method is lately replaced by simplified lens measurement. The photons accumulated for imaging ranged from 14 to 23 Kcounts and the specimen scan time from 10 to 30 min according to the strength of non-decayed residual radioactivity. This low amount of radioactivity was judged to be unhazardous when carefully handled in surgical theater. Scan Image brightness control was done by increasing gamma value up to 95 starting from 50 (the default value) and done and save the finished image with another new name. The use of original naïve digital information and communications in a medicine scan was required as repeatedly mentioned.

On the one hand, conventional radiograph was taken using a standardized radiographic machine and ^{99m}Tc-HDP pinhole bone scan using a gamma camera, Siemens E-cam Signature, Knoxville, ILL, USA. Radiographic exposure factors were 65–70 kVp, 35–40 mAs, and 100 cm source-image distance and the anterior pinhole scan factors were 925–1110 MBq (25–30 mCi) ^{99m}Tc-HDP. On the

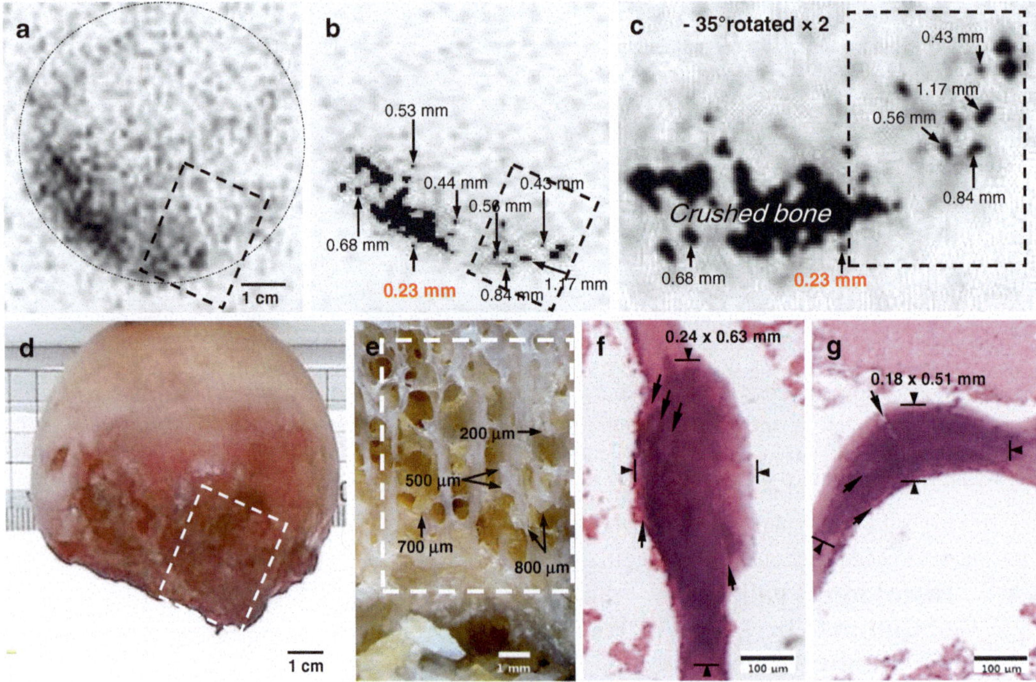

Fig. 6.7 ACDSee-7 gamma correction pinhole bone scan demonstrates callused trabecular microfractures in the femoral neck fracture. (**a**) Naïve pinhole scan of femoral neck fracture shows nonspecific blurry ^{99m}Tc-HDP uptake (frame). (**b**) Gamma correction view shows highlighted mircocalluses (frame). (**c**) Twofold magnified and 35°counterclockwise rotated gamma correction pinhole bone scan shows reoriented gamma correction to closely match with tissue findings. (**d**) Surgically removed specimen. Region of interest marked with frame. (**e**) Surgical microscopic view of the cut surface shows calluses, crushed trabeculae, and normal trabeculae. The smallest microfracture measures 200 μm. (**f, g**) H&E stains show thready microfractures and typical base stain (arrows)

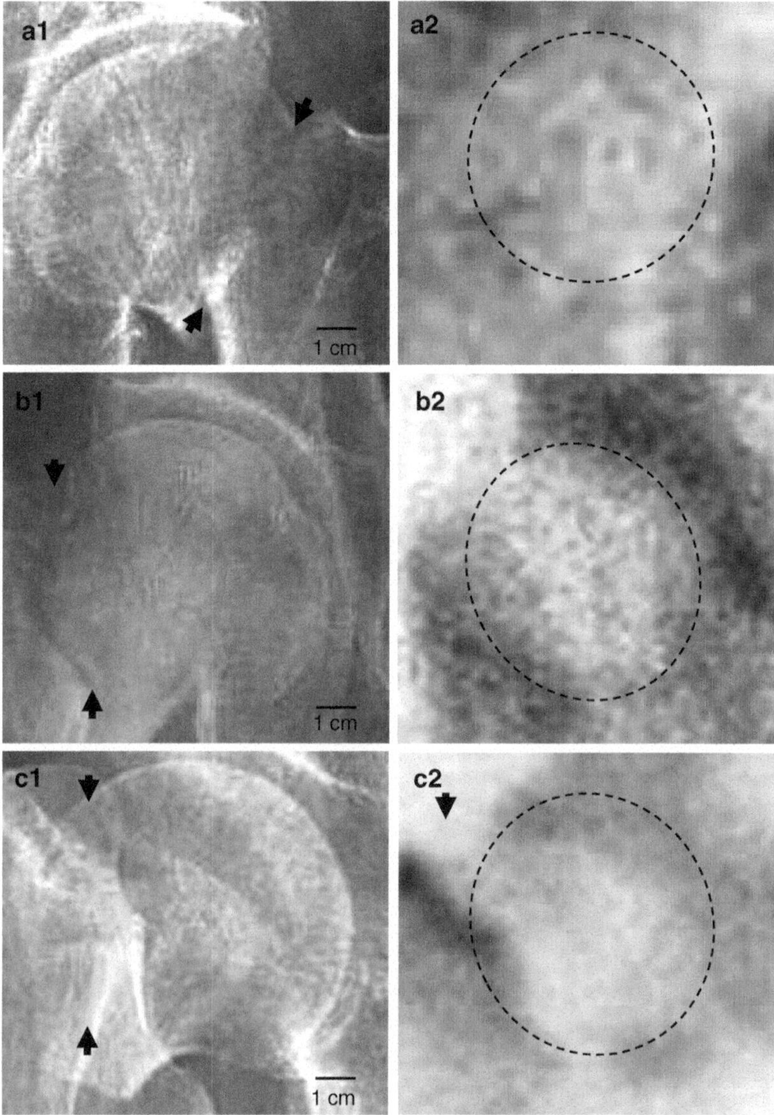

Fig. 6.8 Three different types of femoral neck fracture. Top panel: (**a1**) conventional radiograph in a 74-year-old female shows fracture across the left femoral neck (arrows). Fracture line is indistinct (arrows). (**a2**) Pinhole scan shows photon defect (circle). Intermediary panel: (**b1**) conventional radiograph of the right hip in an 82-year-old male shows fracture across the femoral neck with mild fragment separation (arrows). (**b2**) Pinhole scan shows photon defect in the femoral head (circle). There is reactive tracer uptake in the acetabulum and intertrochanteric zone. Bottom panel: (**c1**) conventional radiograph of the right hip in a 92-year-old male shows fracture in the femoral neck with fragment impaction. (**c2**) ^{99m}Tc-HDP pinhole bone scan shows photon defect in the femoral head (circle) with reactive tracer uptake in femoral tubercle (arrows)

other hand, the femoral head removed by surgery was immediately examined using 4-mm pinhole bone scanning to make advantageous use of receding remnant radionuclide administered to each patient 24 h before surgery. Each of the operatively removed femoral heads was confirmed to reserve a sufficient amount of radioactivity to perform gamma correction scintiscan. In addition, the 10%-formalin cleansed surface of the surgical specimen was scrutinized using surface microscope and confirmed the presence of actively forming callused trabecular microfractures (Fig. 6.7d, e). The processing was then followed by naïve pinhole scanning which showed nonspecific blurry tracer uptake in injured trabeculae (Fig. 6.7a) and subsequently by gamma correction scanning (Fig. 6.7b) which showed distinctly highlighted unsuppressed tracer uptake in the callused trabecular fracture. In this exemplary case, the smallest microcallus measured 230 μm in size. Thereafter, examination was finalized by H&E stain which revealed typical linear microfractures surrounded by purple base stain in calcification (Fig. 6.7f). All these procedures were carried out with strict observation of the radioactivity safety rule. The object bones so analyzed included

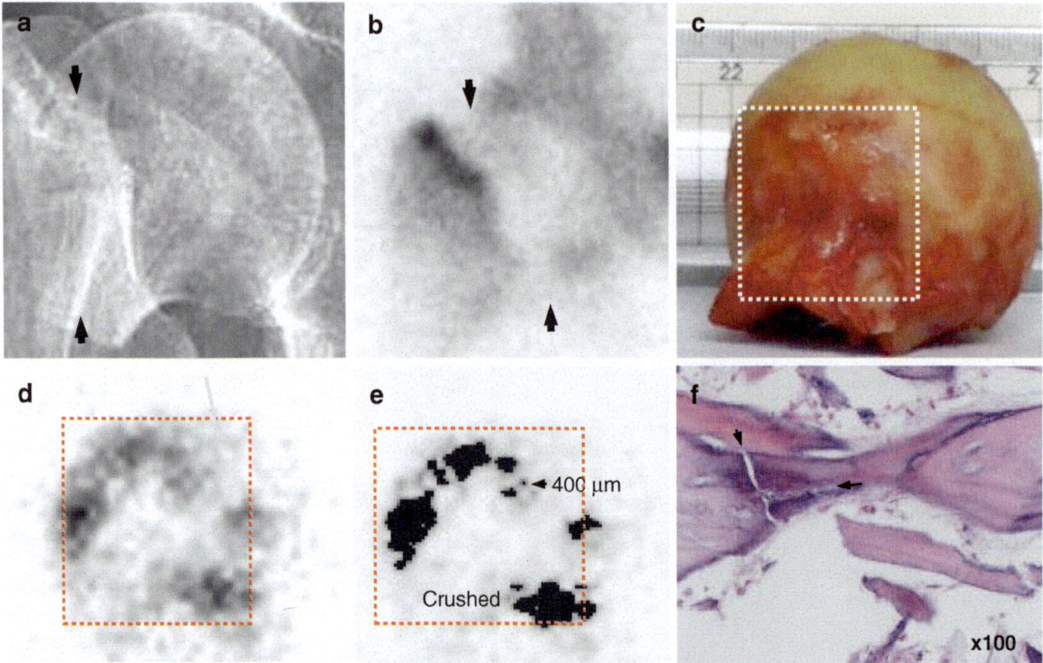

Fig. 6.9 Imaging diagnosis with histological verification of the right femoral neck fracture in a 71-year-old male patient. (**a**) Detailed preoperative conventional radiographic demonstration of a contracted femoral neck fracture. (**b**) Preoperative ^{99m}Tc-HDP pinhole bone scan shows complete photopenia in femoral head. (**c**) Fresh surgical specimen shows fracture with trabecular changes (frame). (**d**, **e**) Naïve and ACDSee-7 gamma correction pinhole scans show nonspecific blurry tracer uptake and unsuppressed tracer uptake in fractures, respectively (frame). The smallest fracture measure 400 µm. (**f**) H&E stain shows lying down T-shaped microfracture with typical base stain in calcification (arrows)

those of the shoulder girdle, hip, and knee. Figure 6.8 shows consolidated results of preoperative conventional radiographs and ^{99m}Tc-HDP pinhole bone scans to show femoral neck fracture and avascular femora-head osteonecrosis. Radiographically, fractures can be scarce and indefinite in appearance, definite with mild separation, or obviously contracted and deformed and photon defect also widely varied in intensity from faint to obvious. Figure 6.9 shows the detailed radiographic demonstration of contracted femoral neck fracture along with naïve and gamma correction pinhole bone scan findings and H&E stain evidence of osteoneogenesis in CTMF. It is to be noted that postoperative imaging studies show only changes which are strictly confined to devascularized or devitalized femoral head and a thereto attached tiny fragmented portion of the femoral neck.

References

Bahk YW. Combined scintigraphic and radiographic diagnosis of bone and joint diseases with gamma correction interpretation. 4th ed. Heidelberg/Berlin: Springer; 2013.

Bahk YW, Jeon HS, Kim JM, et al. A novel use of gamma correction for precise ^{99m}Tc-HDP pinhole bone scan diagnosis and classification of knee occult fractures. Skeletal Radiol. 2010;39:807–81.

Bahk YW, Chung YA, Lee U-Y, et al. Gamma correction ^{99m}hydroxymethylene diphosphante pinhole bone scan diagnosis and histopathological verification of trrabecular contusion in young rats. Nucl Med Commun. 2016;37:988–91.

Bahk YW, Hwang SH, Lee UY, et al. Morphobiochemical diagnosis of acute trabecular microfractures using gamma correction Tc-99m HDP pinhole bone scan with histopathological verification. Medicine. 2017;96(45):e8419.

Fazzarali NL. Trabecular microfracture. Calcif Tissue Int. 1993;53(Suppl 1):S143–6.

Francis MD, Ferguson DL, Tofe AJ, et al. Evaluation of three phosphonates: in vitro adsorption (C-14 labeled) and in vivo osteogenic uptake (Tc-99m complexed). J Nucl Med. 1980;21:1185–9.

Jung JY, Cheon GJ, Lee YS, et al. Pixelized measurement of 99mTc-HDP micro particle formed in gamma correction phantom pinhole scan: a reference study. Nucl Med Mol Imaging. 2016;50:207–12.

Klinstroem SO, Moreno R, Brismar TB. Trabecular bone structure parameters from 3D image processing of clinical multi-slice and cone-beam computed tomography data. Skeletal Radiol. 2014;43: 197–204.

Mandalia V, Henson JH. Traumatic bone bruising—a review article. Eur J Radiol. 2008;67:54–61.

McFarland PH, Frost HL. A possible cause for aseptic necrosis of the femoral head. Henry Ford Med Bull. 1961;9:115–22.

Mink JH, Deutch AL. Occult cartilage and bone injuries of the knee: detection, classification, and assessment with MR imaging. Radiology. 1989;170:823–39.

Rangger C, Kathrein A, Freund MC, et al. Bone bruise of the knee: histology and cryosections in 5 cases. Acta Orthop Scand. 1998;69:291–4.

Ryu KN, Jin W, Ko YT, et al. Bone bruises: MR characteristics and histological correlation in young pig. Clin Imaging. 2000;124:371–80.

Song H, Wehrli. In vivo micro-imaging using alternating navigator echoes with applications to cancellous bone structural analysis. Magn Reson Med. 1999;41:947–53.

Tassani S, Matspoulos GK. The micro-structure of bone trabecular fracture: an inter-city study. Bone. 2014;60:78–6.

Vernon-Roberts B, Pirie CJ. Healing trabecular microfractures in the bodies of lumbar vertebrae. ann Rheum Dis. 1973;32:406–12.

Yao L, Lee JK. Occult intraosseous fracture: detection with MR imaging. Radiology. 1988;170:823–9.

Yoon DK, Jung JY, Hong KJ, et al. Tomographic image of prompt gamma ray from boron neutron capture therapy: a Monte Carlo simulation study. Appl Lett. 2014;105:083521.

Gamma Correction ^{99m}Tc-HDP Pinhole Bone Scan of Callused Trabecular Microfracture in Surgical Specimen: Histological Validation

7

CTMF (callused trabecular microfracture) ubiquitously occurs in osteoporosis (Vernon-Roberts and Pirie 1973), contusion (Mandalia and Henson 2008), aseptic osteonecrosis (McFarland and Frost 1961), inflammatory, metabolic, and neoplastic diseases of bone (Bahk 2017) and even normal physiological activity (Fazzarali 1993; Frost 1973). Its clinical effect may be negligible when localized but once widespread or systemic, it may become a serious disease to disturb the equilibrium state of whole skeletal system manifesting not only as a major debilitating disease but also as a serious welfare and socioeconomic problem, especially in aged population (Tassani and Matsopoulos 2013). CTMF heals by producing callus, an aggregation of woven bone, manifesting as a "nodular, fusiform, angulated, or arched bridge lesion" (Fazzarali 1993) (Fig. 7.1a). Pinhole scan demonstrates avid tracer accumulation in CTMF, which was not suppressed by gamma correction (Fig. 7.1b). The adjective of "callus" is "callused" meaning "covered with callus" (Webster's New International Dictionary, Unabridged).

Devascularized necrotic femoral head is to be removed by surgery to perform arthroplasty. For this gamma correction study, six consecutive patients were recruited with their consent after the diagnostic confirmation of osteonecrosis of the femoral head due to femoral neck fracture and surgical specimen was examined using ^{99m}Tc-HDP pinhole bone scanning (Fig. 7.2). First, fractured surfaces shown on femoral head specimen of all patients was individually scrutinized using a surgical microscope to confirm and record already formed seed-pearly calluses. Then, the microscopic findings were meticulously correlated with the findings of GCPBS and H&E stain in each case for histological confirmation. As anticipated, the size and shape of damaged trabeculae shown on GCPBS varied from pinpointed to large irregular archipelagic lesions and occasionally some of pinpointed trabecular microfractures needed magnification for accurate assay (Fig. 7.3b, c). Regardless of size and shape the radioactivity detected in those microfractures were derived from residua of ^{99m}Tc-HDP, which was intravenously administered to patients for one-day preoperative bone scanning. Technically, the amount of radiotracer, aperture-to-object distance, field of view size, and matrix size were 1.0–1.07 GBq (3.7–4.0 mCi), 12 cm, 14 x 14 cm, and 256 × 256, respectively. Those data were needed for the mathematical calculation of pixelized measurement (Jung et al. 2016). The number of photons

Y.-W. Bahk, *Imaging of Trabecular Microfracture and Bone Marrow Edema and Hemorrhage*,
https://doi.org/10.1007/978-981-15-4466-8_7

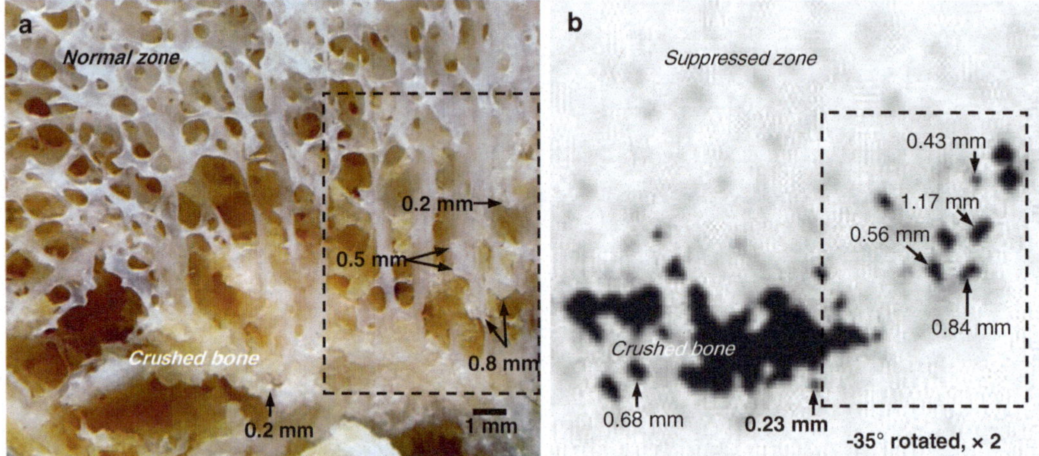

Fig. 7.1 Surgical microscopic view of cut surface and validating gamma correction ^{99m}Tc-HDP pinhole bone scan. (**a**) Surgical surface microscopy shows callused microfractures and crushed trabeculae (frame) as well as normal trabeculae. (**b**) Twofold magnified gamma correction pinhole bone scan demonstrates unsuppressed tracer uptake, which is same-looking crushed and pinpointed callused microtrabeculae (frame). The smallest microfractures measure 0.2 mm (200 μm) on a microscope and 0.23 mm (230 μm) on gamma correction pinhole scan (Jung et al. 2016), respectively

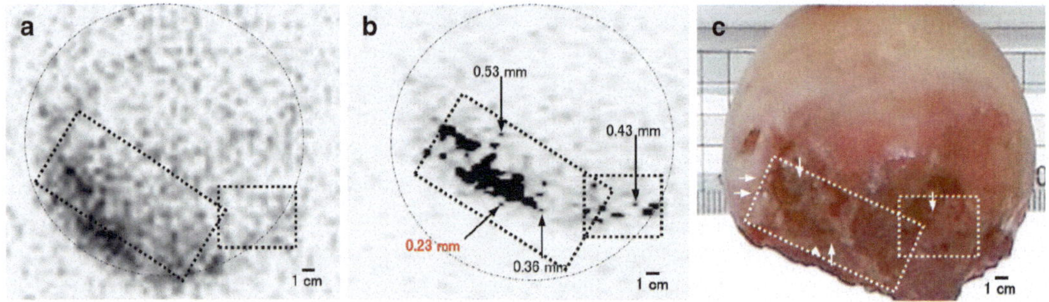

Fig. 7.2 Precise demonstration and quantitation of callused trabecular microfractures in femoral neck fracture in a 72-year-old female patient using visuospatial–mathematical assay (Bahk et al. 2019). (**a**) Naïve pinhole scan of femoral neck shows nonspecific blurry tracer uptake (square frames). (**b**) Gamma correction suppresses edema and hemorrhage uptake neatly highlighting callused microfractures the size of which was measured using pixelized measurement (Jung et al. 2016). (**c**) Fresh surgical specimen shows microfractures (arrows) and archipelagic crushed bones (square frames)

accumulated for pinhole scan ranged from 14 to 23 Kilocounts and scan time ranged from 10 to 30 min according to the strength of undecayed residual radioactivity. Image brightness control was achieved by increasing gamma value up to 95 starting from 50 (default value) and "done" and "save" keys were pushed to finish gamma correction with the last new name. As mentioned, gamma correction pinhole scan image can be properly magnified to accommodate the observer's eyesight (Fig. 7.3c). Figure 7.4 is another case presenting a femoral neck fracture in a 92-year-old-male patient. He fell down from sleeping bed onto the uncarpeted floor.

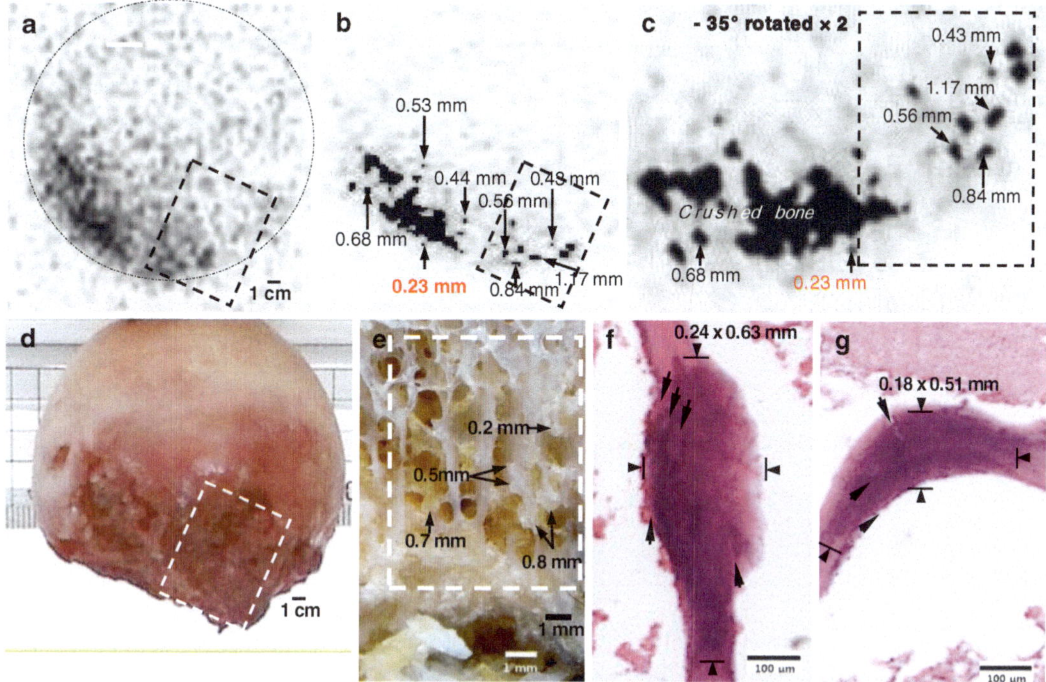

Fig. 7.3 Gamma correction pinhole bone scan distinctly demonstrates trabecular microcalluses in femoral neck fracture. (**a**) Naïve pinhole scan of femoral neck fracture shows blurry fractures due to edema and hemorrhage (frame). (**b**) Gamma correction view shows highlighted mircocalluses (frame). (**c**) Twofold magnified and 35° counterclockwise rotated gamma correction pinhole bone scan shows reoriented gamma correction to match with tissue findings. (**d**) Surgically removed specimen. Region of interest marked with frame. (**e**) Surgical microscopic view of the cut surface shows calluses, crushed trabeculae, and normal trabeculae. The smallest callus measures 0.2 mm or 200 μm. (**f, g**) H&E stains show thready microfractures and typical base stain (arrows)

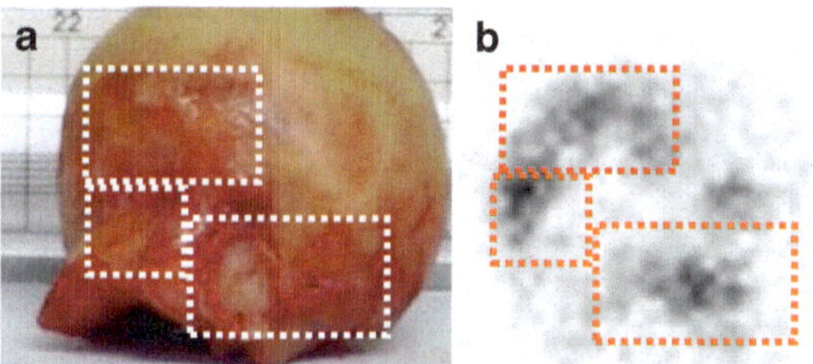

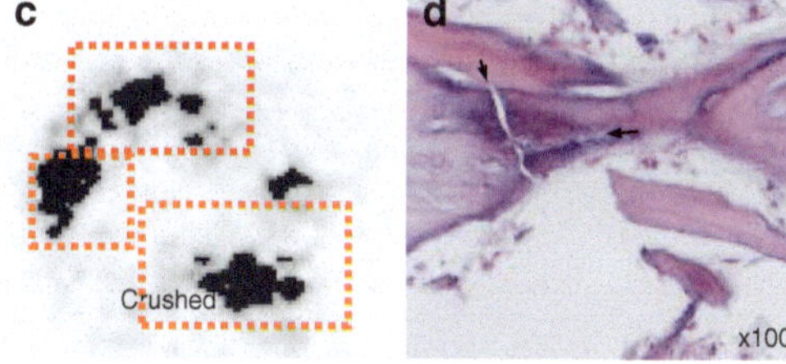

Fig. 7.4 Right femoral neck fracture in a 92-year-old-male. (**a**) Fresh surgical specimen shows femoral neck fracture and ROIs in the neck portion of the femoral head (frames). (**b**) Naïve pinhole scan shows nonspecific blurry tracer uptake areas (frames). (**c**) Gamma correction pinhole scan shows crushed fractures. (**d**) H&E stain shows lying-down T-shaped fracture with calcification (arrows)

References

Bahk YW. Combined scintigraphic and radiographic diagnosis of bone and joint diseases with gamma correction interpretation. 5th ed. Heidelberg/Berlin: Springer; 2017.

Bahk YW, Kim EE, Chung YA, et al. Precise differential diagnosis of acute bone marrow edema and hemorrhage and trabecular microfractures using naïve and gamma correction pinhole bone scans. J Internat Med Research. 2019. https://doi.org/10.1177/0300060518819910.

Fazzarali NL. Trabecular microfracture. Calcif Tissue Int. 1993;53(Suppl 1):S143–6.

Frost HM. The spinal osteoporosis. Mechanisms of pathogenesis and pathophysiology. Clin Endocrinol Metab. 1973;2:257–75.

Jung JY, Cheon GJ, Lee YS, et al. Pixelized measurement of 99mTc-HDP micro particle formed in gamma correction phantom pinhole scan: a reference study. Nucl Med Mol Imaging. 2016;50:207–12.

Mandalia V, Henson JH. Traumatic bone bruising—a review article. Eur J Radiol. 2008;67:54–61.

McFarland PH, Frost HL. A possible cause for aseptic necrosis of the femoral head. Henry Ford Med Bull. 1961;9:115–22.

Tassani S, Matsopoulos GK. The micro-structure of bone trabecular fracture: an inter-site study. Bone. 2013;60:78–86.

Vernon-Roberts B, Pirie CJ. Healing trabecular microfractures in the bodies of lumbar vertebrae. Ann Rheum Dis. 1973;32:406–12.

8 Mathematic and Magnifying Lens Measurements of ^{99m}Tc-HDP Uptake in Callused Trabecular Microfracture

Recently, we developed two kinds of different size-measurement method of the ^{99m}Tc-HDP uptake in CTMF. One is the mathematic size quantitation of micro-uptake formed in a gamma correction pinhole scan phantom (Jung et al. 2016) and the other one is direct counting of the number of pixel(s) affected with trabecular microfracture on ACDSee-10 gamma correction pinhole bone scan using a 10× magnifying optic lens.

8.1 Mathematic Calculation of Micro ^{99m}Tc-HDP Uptake Size

The size of individual micro ^{99m}Tc HDP uptake was mathematically calculated using the pixelized measurement method (Fig. 8.1) (Jung et al. 2016). Each micro-spot was appointed as a region of interest (ROI). The image profile is presented in a line spread function denoting the signal intensity of the applied line. The *Y*-axis of the image profile is signal intensity and the *X*-axis shows the pixel number in profile. In order to easily measure the full width at half maximum (FWHM), matrix size was expanded to 512 × 512. Because of the increased number of pixels, the signal intensity value was assigned by interpolation at the expanded bin which does not have a signal intensity value. To interpolate the between bins, the Gaussian curve fitting method was used using the in-house MATLAB code (Mathworks, R2011a, USA) (Jung et al. 2016). The equation of the Gaussian curve fitting was as below:.

$$y(x) = \frac{1}{\sigma\sqrt{2\pi}} \exp\left[-\frac{(x - x_0)^2}{2\sigma}\right]$$

y = interpolated value
x = original frame value
x_0 = mean value of the frame value
σ = standard deviation

The micrographic ^{99m}Tc-HDP deposits used in this study were naturally formed in the water-flooded phantom into which ^{99m}Tc-HDP was injected (Fig. 8.1a, b). Such deposit formation was found accidentally by the corresponding author. The acrylic planar phantom we used was Model 043-054 of Biodex Medical Systems Inc., Shirley, New York, USA. Its dimension was 52 × 71.1 × 3.2 cm. To begin with, the phantom was flooded with 3000 ml of distilled water and 370 MBq (10 mCi) of ^{99m}Tc-HDP were therein injected through an injection port. The phantom was then gently shaken manually for 20 min to diffuse and homogenize the tracer injected in the floodwater. Despite the shaking, however, naturally tracer deposits formed along the tracer injection trail. Deposits thus created were too small to see with unaided eyes needing magnification using 4-mm pinhole scanning for accurate sized measurement. Two hundred Kcounts were accumulated in 10 min.

Y.-W. Bahk, *Imaging of Trabecular Microfracture and Bone Marrow Edema and Hemorrhage*,
https://doi.org/10.1007/978-981-15-4466-8_8

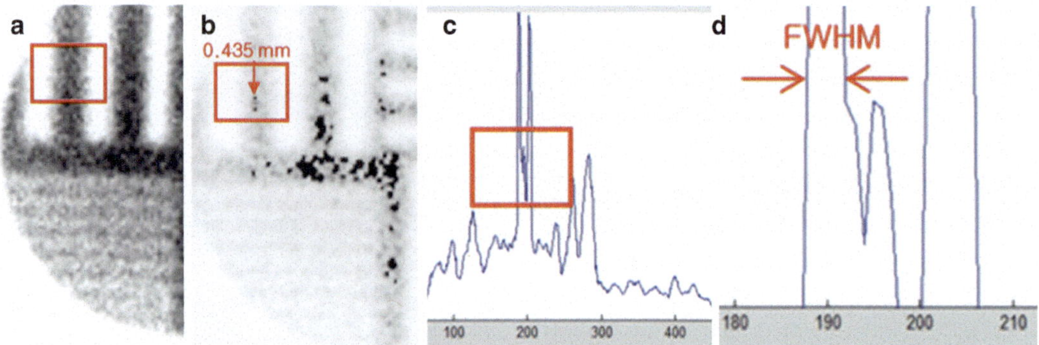

Fig. 8.1 Effect of gamma correction experimentally tested using a bar flood phantom. (**a**) Naïve pinhole scan shows unmeasurable nebulous radioactivity of ^{99m}Tc-HDP (frame). (**b**) ACDSee-7 gamma correction view of ROI clearly discerns ^{99m}Tc-HDP deposits so that their size can be calculated using pixelized measurement. (**c**) Pixelized measurement of smaller vertical profile is extracted from ROI (red frame). (**d**) Enlarged view of the ROI in profile. Two points are picked to calculate FWHM (Jung et al. 2016)

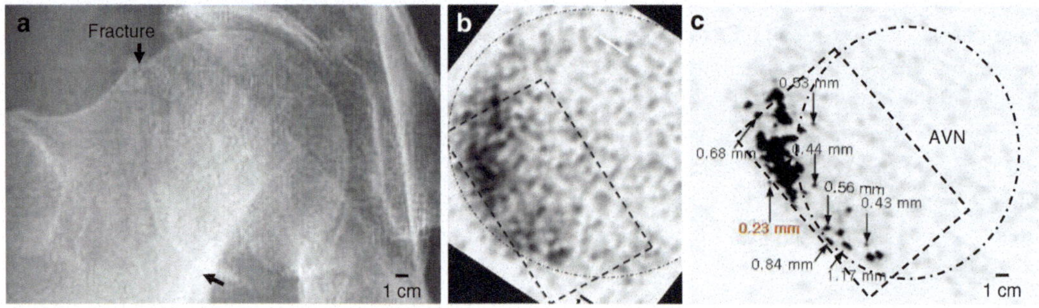

Fig. 8.2 Faint femoral neck fracture in a 37-year-old male due to motor vehicle accident. (**a**) Anteroposterior radiograph of the right hip shows faint curved linear fracture across the femoral neck (arrows). The femoral head is circled. (**b**) Naïve ^{99m}Tc-HDP pinhole bone scan shows nonspecific blurry tracer uptake (frame). (**c**) Gamma correction view shows suppression of edema and highlighted trabecular fractures with the smallest one measuring 0.23 mm (or 230 μm). AVN denotes avascular necrosis

In the meantime, a clinical application study of this mathematic quantitation method was performed in six patients including 3 males and 3 females with the age ranging from 72 to 92 years with a mean being 78.4 years (Bahk et al. 2017). The causes of femoral neck fracture were falling down from a bed or chair, slipping in staircase, or tumbling in toilet or street. The preoperative anatomical diagnosis of femoral fracture was made in each patient using conventional radiography (Fig. 8.2a) and the avascular necrosis was confirmed by ^{99m}Tc-HDP pinhole bone scan. It was then followed by naïve and gamma correction pinhole bone scans to confirm the avascular necrosis of the femoral head and to demonstrate callused trabecular microfractures formed in the vascularized distal half of the fractured femoral neck (Fig. 8.2b, c). On the day next, the necrotized femoral head with a portion of the subcapital neck was removed by surgery to perform arthroplasty. Surgical specimen was assessed immediately after resection using a surface microscope to confirm that callused trabecular microfractures were already formed (Fig. 8.3c, d) and finally the specimen was histologically assessed using H&E staining histologically confirming trabecular microfractures (Fig. 8.3e). The injured surface of each specimen was cleansed and scrutinized using a surface microscope to assure that microcalluses were formed and anatomical findings of microcalluses were conclusively compared with those of GCPBS and H&E

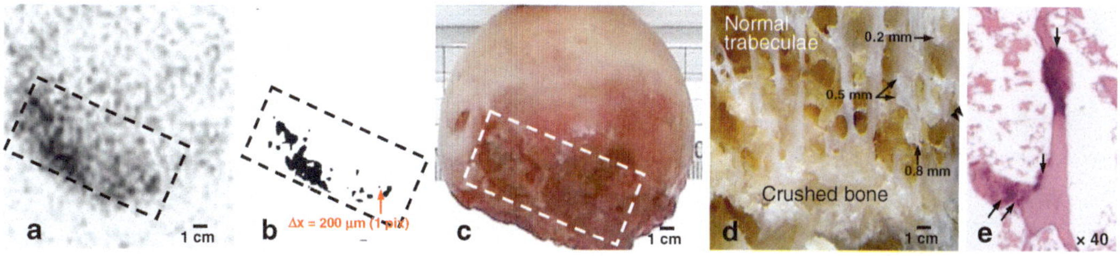

Fig. 8.3 ACDSee-10 gamma correction pinhole bone scan demonstration and quantitation of callused trabecular microfractures. (**a**) Naïve pinhole scan shows blurry ^{99m}Tc-HDP uptake in edematous microcalluses (frame). (**b**) Upgraded ACDSee-10 gamma correction pinhole bone scan suppresses edema and hemorrhage uptake highlighting microcallus, which measures 200 μm in size consisting of a single pixel. (**c**) Surgical specimen shows microcalluses in femoral neck (frame). (**d**) Surgical surface microscopy shows callused trabecular microfractures and crushed bone as well as normal trabeculae. (**e**) H&E stain shows microfractures with base stain (arrows)

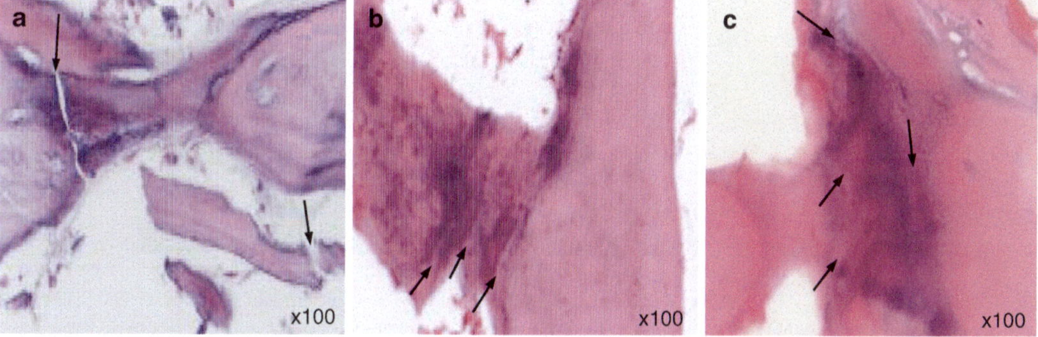

Fig. 8.4 Trabecular microfractures can be variously defined on H&E stain. It can be sharply defined (**a**), intermediary defined (**b**), and blurry defined (**c**). Regardless of fracture demonstration base H&E stain reflects osteoneogenesis

stain for histological validation (Fig. 8.2). Callused microfractures were presented as fine whitish thready shadows surrounded by basophilic matrix (Fig. 8.4). Fractures were sharply, intermediately, or undefinedly delineated. Some were meshy and granular in appearance. All these tests were performed carefully observing the regulation of preventive radiation hazards although the amount of the radiotracer therein used was negligible. As shown in Fig. 8.1, we first used a Photo Correction Wizard program of ACDSee-7 Photo Editor (ACD systems, Miami, FL (Bahk et al. 2017) for the measurement of microcalluses, but, as mentioned above, more recently we shifted it to upgraded ACDSee 10 in which the size of microcallus was more correctly measured using magnifying lens because pixels were now very neatly imaged without penumbra as shown in Fig. 8.5. This improved penumbra-free image permitted us to accurately measure the microfracture using a simple optic lens not bothering mathematic calculation because the accurate size of callused trabecular microfracture can now be measured simply using an optic lens in terms of pixel involvement.

8.2 Magnifying Lens Measurement of ^{99m}Tc-HDP Uptake Size on Gamma Correction Pinhole Bone Scan and H&E Stain Patterns

Figure 8.6a is the photograph of a fresh femoral head operatively removed to perform arthroplasty. The specimen retained some minimal undecayed residual tracer which renders specimen scan possible. Naïve pinhole bone scan (Fig. 8.6b) of the surgical specimen shows irregular areas of nonspecific nebulous ^{99m}Tc-HDP

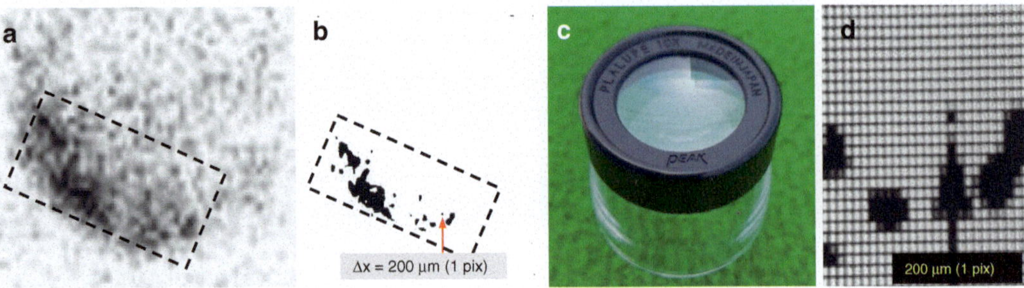

Fig. 8.5 Gamma correction ^{99m}Tc-HDP pinhole bone scan demonstration and quantitation of 200 μm microcallus formed in trabecular fracture. (**a**) Naïve pinhole scan of the right femoral neck fracture shows nonspecific tracer uptake in callused trabecular microfractures which were blurred due to edema and hemorrhage (frame). (**b**) ACDSee-10 gamma correction highlights single-pixeled 200 μm microcallus. Δx is the x-axis. (**c**) Tenfold magnifying lens. (**d**) Close-up view of single pixel microcallus taken by a built-in camera cell phone (Galaxy Note 8, Samsung, Seoul)

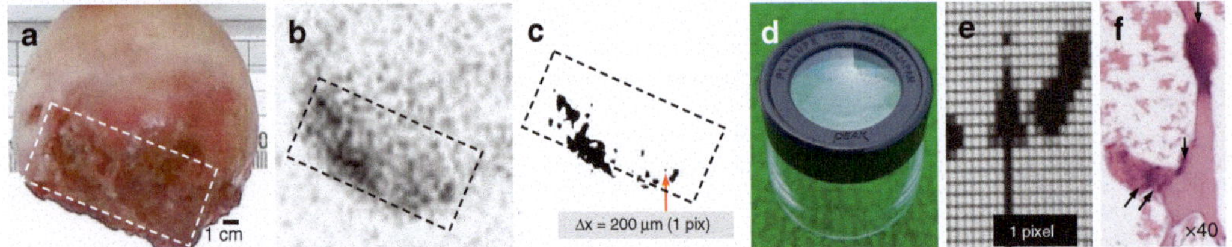

Fig. 8.6 Gamma correction ^{99m}Tc-HDP pinhole bone scan can neatly demonstrate single-pixel trabecular microfracture which measures 200 μm in size using an ordinary magnifying lens. (**a**) Fresh surgical specimen shows microfractures formed in femoral neck fracture surface (*frame*). (**b**) Naïve coronal pinhole scan shows nonspecific blurry tracer uptake. (**c**) In contrast, ACDSsee-10 gamma correction view can highlight single-pixel 200-μm microfracture (*arrow*). Δx is the x-axis. (**d**) 10× magnifying optic lens. (**e**) Magnified view of ROI shows typical one-pixel involvement. One pixel measures 200 μm. (**f**) H&E stain shows base stained microcalluses. This presentation proves that the accurate size of callused trababecular microfracture can be precisely measured using a magnifying lens

uptake of various intensities. The shape and size of such nebulous uptake cannot be assessed in any detail, but gamma correction suppresses the nebulous uptake of edema and hemorrhage now very neatly highlighting microfractures without any penumbra (Fig. 8.6c). The size of individual microfracture needs image magnification for accurate size measurement using an ordinary magnification lens (Fig. 8.6d). The smallest microcallus so measured in this case was 200 μm in size. The surface microscopic findings of seed-pearly microcalluses and crushed bone were in good accord with the pinpoint and crushed bone tracer uptake in GCPBS. H&E stain showed injured basophilic trabeculae in bone marrow along with fat cell deposition, fibrosis, edema, and hemorrhage (Fig. 8.6f). It is thus well confirmed that gamma correction can uniquely and specifically demonstrate trabecular microfractures (Fig. 8.6e). As mentioned all these nuclear bone imaging procedures were performed strictly observing the safety rule of radiation hazard. Indeed, the radiation dose per se was within the safety range. Actually, radiation is much less than routine clinical bone scanning through 24-h physical decay.

References

Bahk YW, Hwang SH, Lee UY, et al. Morphobiochemical diagnosis of acute trabecular microfractures using gamma correction Tc-99m HDP pinhole bone scan with histopathological verification. Medicine. 2017;96(45):e8419.

Jung JY, Cheon GJ, Lee YS, et al. Pixelized measurement of 99mTc-HDP micro particle formed in gamma correction phantom pinhole scan: a reference study. Nucl Med Mol Imaging. 2016;50:207–12.

9 Corroborative Analysis of Callused Trabecular Microfracture on ^{99m}Tc-HDP Pinhole Bone Scan, Surgical Specimen, GCPBS, and H&E Stain

As anticipated the shape and size of trabecular fracture widely vary presenting as pinpoint, speckle, rod-like, archipelagic, geographic, and amorphously crushed tracer uptake. Indeed, some are large and some are pinpointed in size and some are numerous and some are scanty (Fig. 9.1). Fortunately, however, the scrutiny and correlation of findings demonstrated in the surgical specimen and surface microscope (Fig. 9.2), naïve and gamma correction pinhole scans (Fig. 9.3), and H&E stain (Fig. 9.4) were all in good accord. Practically, the conventional radiograph, fresh surgical specimen, naïve and gamma correction pinhole bone scans, surgical microscope, and H&E stain consistently showed neck fracture, femoral head surface injury, nebulous tracer uptake, distinct microfracture uptake, seed-pearly microcallus, and whitish thready and meshy microfractures with typical basophilic H&E stain, respectively. Basically, all these findings were considered to be due to calcifying callus, which is actively engaged with trabecular microfracture healing. GCPBS can accurately diagnose microfractures with pinpoint, speckled, rod-like, and geometric ^{99m}Tc-HDP uptake along with archipelagic crushed trabeculae. Furthermore, GCPBS highlights actively forming trabecular fractures with enhanced tracer uptake, which is characteristically unsuppressed by gamma correction. The ^{99m}Tc-HDP uptake in reactive endosteal rimming induced in rats by falling iron ball contusion also showed the same change with unsuppressed tracer uptake (Bahk et al. 2017). Thus, it has been fully confirmed that ACDSee 10 gamma correction can efficiently demonstrate trabecular fractures including microfractures, one of which measures 200 μm in size. The demonstrability of microfractures may vary according to not only the physical nature of the trauma or stress but also to the type of ACDSee gamma correction used. Indeed, it may be scanty, moderate, or multiple or even countless due to the different grade of causative trauma and the corrected image can be blurry or sharp according to the version of the gamma correction used (Fig. 9.1). Old ACDSee-7 version gamma correction (Fig. 9.1a, b) suffers from blurry penumbra, but it can be rectified simply when the upgraded ACDSee 10 is used (Fig. 9.1c).

Clinically, callused microfractures ubiquitously occur in a large variety of bone diseases (Vernon-Roberts and Pirie 1973; Mandalia and Henson 2008; McFarland and Frost 1961; Bahk et al. 2016; Fazzarali 1993) and even in normal physiological activity (Frost 1973; Tassani and Matsopoulos 2014). CTMF is the micro breakage of trabeculae, which measures approximately 0.5 mm in thickness (Vernon-Roberts, Pirie

Y.-W. Bahk, *Imaging of Trabecular Microfracture and Bone Marrow Edema and Hemorrhage*,
https://doi.org/10.1007/978-981-15-4466-8_9

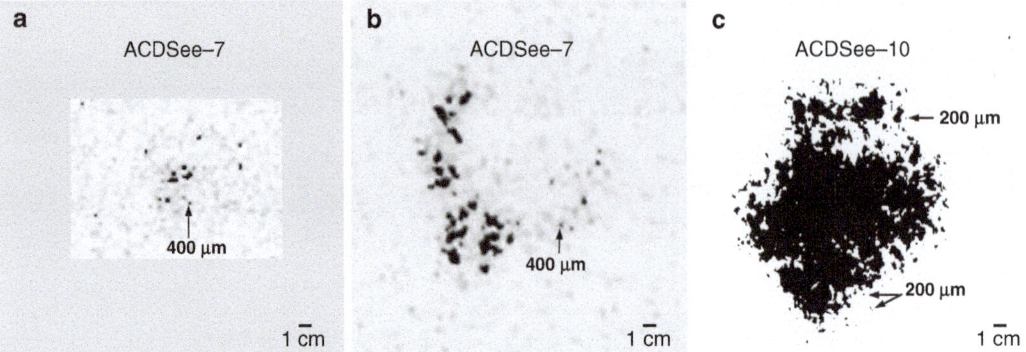

Fig. 9.1 Scanty, multiple, and numerous presentations of trabecular fractures are demonstrated by gamma correction ^{99m}Tc-HDP pinhole bone scan in three different patients. (**a**, **b**) ACDSee-7 gamma correction pinhole scan was used in the first and second cases showing scanty and multiple callused microfractures that are unfortunately blurry in appearance because of penumbra. (**c**) In contrast, however, the upgraded ACDSee-10 gamma correction neatly suppresses the penumbra sharply demonstrating microfractures that are numerous and uncountable. The smallest ones measure 200 μm in size (arrow)

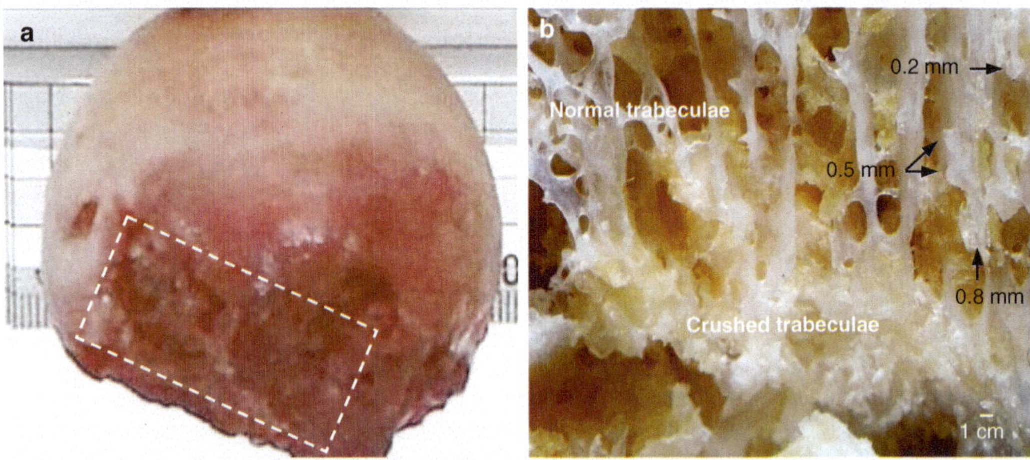

Fig. 9.2 Fresh surgical specimen and surgical surface microscopic findings. (**a**) Surgical specimen shows roughened fracture surface including microcalluses. (**b**) Surgical microscopic view of cut surface shows calluses, crushed trabeculae, and normal trabeculae. The smallest fracture measures 0.2 mm (or 200 μm) in size

1973) and heals by callus formation. The callus is a micronodular aggregate of woven bone and typically looks like a seed pearl (Fig. 9.2b). GCPBS is currently used for the microanatomical diagnosis of occult fractures and other bone diseases (Bahk et al. 2016). Besides, bone contusion incites endoblastic rimming to repair trabecular injury as confirmed by rat experiment (Bahk et al. 2016). Gamma correction can distinguish the normal bone with mild ^{99m}Tc- HDP uptake and the edema and hemorrhage dipped bone with intermediate uptake from the actively forming callus with highly enhanced tracer uptake in fractured or bruised trabeculae. Such biochemically different suppression of ^{99m}Tc-HDP uptake appears to be helpful for the differential diagnosis of edema, hemorrhage, microfracture, or trabecular bruise. Recognizing the ever increasing clinical and socioeconomic importance of trabecular microfracture new imaging tools are being actively developed including micro-CT (Okazaki et al. 2014) and multislice cone-beam

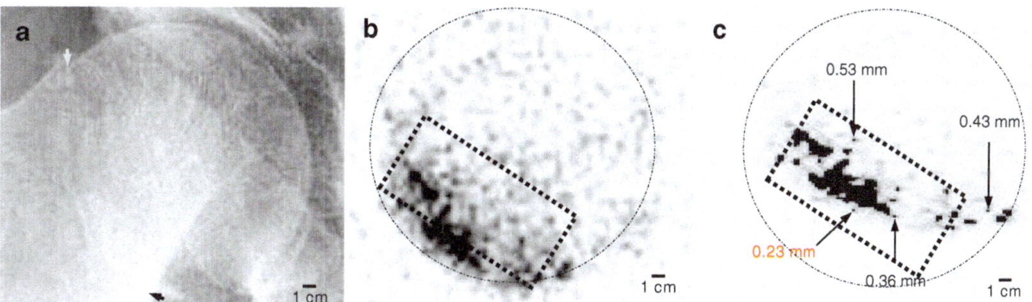

Fig. 9.3 Visuospatial-mathematic assay (VSMA) can precisely visualize, diagnose, and quantify microcalluses and edema and hemorrhage (Bahk et al. 2019) in femoral neck fracture. The assay consists of seriated naïve and gamma correction pinhole bone scans, pixel size measurement, and NIH ImageJ densitometry. (**a**) Radiographic demonstration of femoral neck fracture. (**b**) Naïve pinhole scan of femoral neck shows nonspecific blurry fractures (frame). (**c**) Gamma correction highlights microcallus and the size of callus can be measured using pixelized measurement. The smallest one measures 0.23 mm or 230 μm in size

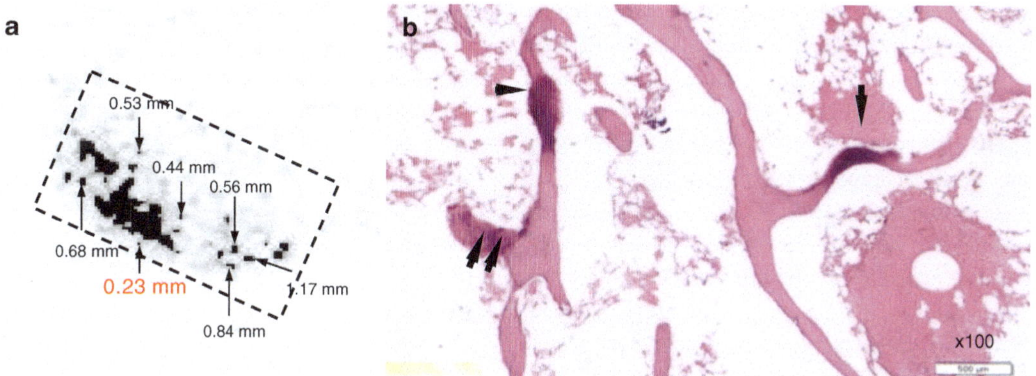

Fig. 9.4 Characteristic trabecular micro and archipelagic fractures. (**a**) Gamma correction pinhole bone scan shows highlighted microcalluses and archipelagic trabecular macrofractures (frame). The smallest callus measures 0.23 mm or 230 μm by arithmetic pixel calculation. (**b**) H&E stain of the same case shows three microcalluses. Two are fusiform in shape and one is multilinear with classic base stain. Observe marrow edema and hemorrhage as well as fat replacement

CT (Klinstrom et al. 2014) and micro-MRI (Rajapakse et al. 2012).

We performed combined bone scan imaging-histology study for two reasons using fresh surgical specimens of traumatically devascularized femoral head in patients. The first reason was to histologically prove that GCPBS can precisely visualize and identify CTMF. The second reason was to biochemically support that gamma correction can efficiently suppress the ^{99m}Tc-HDP uptake in normal bone and edema and hemorrhage and conversely preserves the enhanced high tracer uptake in CTMF. The results of our study indicate that GCPBS can precisely identify calcifying trabecular microfractures and the high tracer uptake in them is not suppressed by gamma correction (Fig. 9.3).

The size of the microcallus can be measured using pixelized method (Yoon et al. 2015; Jung et al. 2016) and also using a magnifying optic lens (Vide Chap. 11, Bahk et al. 2019). The function is an image profile that shows the signal intensity from image matrix. Actually, the size was calculated by measuring the full width at half maximum (FWHM) of the signal peak. The results of our gamma correction study revealed that the pinpoint and otherwise shaped ^{99m}Tc-HDP uptake shown by surface photomicrography

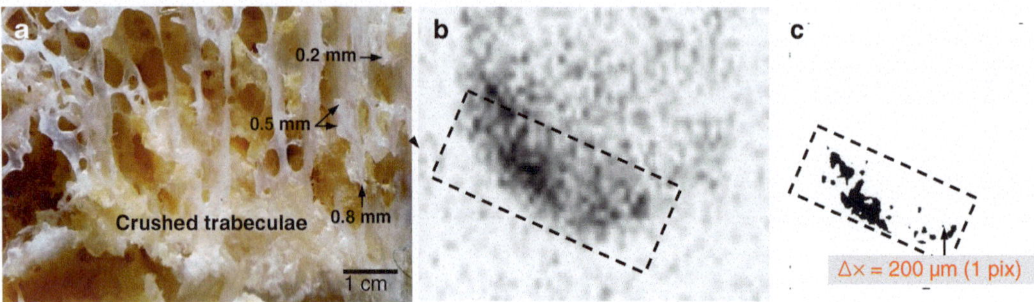

Fig. 9.5 The results of the gamma correction ^{99m}Tc-HDP pinhole bone scan imaging of pinpoint and otherwise shaped uptake in trabecular microfractures as demonstrated on surface photomicrograph. (**a**) Surface photomicrograph of surgically resected femoral neck fracture shows actively ongoing seed-pearly callused trabecular microfracture. (**b**) Naïve ^{99m}Tc-HDP pinhole bone scan shows nonspecific blurry tracer uptake in traumatized trabeculae (frame). (**c**) ACDSee-10 gamma correction shows neatly defined archipelagic and pinpointed microfractures with the smallest one measuring 200 μm (one pixel) in size

and GCPBS (Fig. 9.5) is in good accord proving that the micro ^{99m}Tc-HDP uptake in GCPBS is nothing but ongoing callus formation. Furthermore, the extended correlation of findings of GCPBS, surgical microscope, and H&E stain showed good agreement.

In order to image trabecular microfractures, synchrotron radiation micro CT was devised by Okazaki et al. (2014) obtaining a 3D image of the microcallus in TMF in osteoporotic femoral head as we did in the current experiment. Our series was exclusively focused on the individual callused trabecular microfracture that is distinctly imaged with unsuppressed high ^{99m}Tc-HDP uptake. It is to be pointed out that the ^{99m}Tc-HDP pinhole scan of trabecular microfracture is specifically focused on CTMF, whereas the synchrotron radiation micro-CT visualizes trabeculae and rough callus together as quantification unit. A strong radiobiochemical advantage of GCPBS is that it can uniquely provide bone metabolic profile of CTMF enabling one to qualitatively and quantitatively assess the healing of the callus in microfracture.

In conclusion, GCPBS can be advantageously used for the morphological and radiobiochemical diagnosis of CTMF. The smallest microfracture shown in this study was 230 μm in size when pixelization method is used (Jung et al. 2016) and 200 μm when magnifying lens is used. GCPBS can distinguish CTMF with highly enhanced unsuppressed ^{99m}Tc-HDP uptake from the intact and edema or hemorrhage dipped trabeculae with cleanly suppressed tracer uptake. This method is easy to perform and economical providing us with an important morphobiochemical profile in actively healing trabecular microfracture.

References

Bahk YW, Chung YA, Lee UY, Park SI. Gamma correction 99mTc-hydroymethylene diphosphonate pinhole bone scan diagnosis and histological verification of trabecular contusion in rats. Nucl Med Commun. 2016;7:988–91.

Bahk YW, Hwang SH, Lee UY, et al. Morphobiochemical diagnosis of acute trabecular microfractures using gamma correction Tc-99m HDP pinhole bone scan with histopathological verification. Medicine. 2017;96(45):e8419.

Bahk YW, Kim EE, Chung YA, et al. Precise differential diagnosis of acute bone marrow edema and hemorrhage and trabecular microfractures using naïve and gamma correction pinhole scans. J Int Med Res. 2019; https://doi.org/10.1177/0300060518819910.

Fazzarali NL. Trabecular microfracture. Calcif Tissue Int. 1993;53(Suppl 1):S143–6.

Frost HM. The spinal osteoporosis. Mechanisms of pathogenesis and pathophysiology. Clin Endocrinol Metab. 1973;2:257–75.

Jung JY, Cheon GJ, Lee YS, et al. Pixelized measurement of 99mTc-HDP micro particle formed in gamma correction phantom pinhole scan: a reference study. Nucl Med Mol Imaging. 2016;50:207–12.

Klinstrom E, Smedby O, Moreno R, et al. Trabecular bone structure parameter from 3D image processing of clinical multi-slice and cone-beam computed tomography data. Skelet Radiol. 2014;43:197–204.

Mandalia V, Henson JH. Traumatic bone bruising—a review article. Eur J Radiol. 2008;67:54–61.

McFarland PH, Frost HM. A possible cause for aseptic necrosis of the femoral head. Henry Ford Hospital Med Bulletin. 1961;9:115–22.

Okazaki N, Chiba K, Taguchi K, et al. Trabecular microfractures in the femoral head with osteoporosis: analysis of microcallus formations by synchrotron radiation micro CT. Bone. 2014;64:82–67.

Rajapakse CS, Leonard MB, Bhagat YA, et al. Micro-MR imaging-based computational biomechanics demonstrates reduction in cortical and trabecular bone strength after renal transplantation. Radiology. 2012;262:912–20.

Tassani S, Matsopoulos GK. The micro-structure of bone trabecular fracture: an inter-site study. Bone. 2014;60:78–86.

Vernon-Roberts B, Pirie CJ. Healing trabecular microfractures in the bodies of lumbar vertebrae. Ann Rheum Dis. 1973;32:406–12.

Yoon DK, Jung JY, Han SM, et al. Statistical analysis for discrimination of prompt gamma ray peak induced by high energy neutron: monte Carlo smulation study. 2015;303:859–66.

10 ACDSee-10 Gamma Correction ^{99m}Tc-HDP Pinhole Bone Scan of Normal Adult Bone Skeleton Viewed from the Stand Point of Wolff's Law

Julius Wolff stated in 1892 that "Every change in the form and function of bone or of their function alone is followed by certain definite changes in their internal architecture, and equally definite alteration in their external conformation in accordance with mathematical laws." (Wolff 1892; Alexander and Elma 2016). His statement was highlighted in his monograph, "Das Gesetz der Transformation von Knochen," not an article in a journal. According to a medical dictionary his statement is currently paraphrased as a bone, normal or abnormal, develops the structure most suited to resist the forces acting upon it (Dorland's Illustrated Medical Dictionary, 32nd edition by Elsevier Saunders 2012, p. 1011). We first tentatively checked if there is any significant difference exists among the ACDsee-10 gamma correction values in the cervical, thoracic, and lumbar spines finding that the gamma values were 85 in the normal cervical and thoracic spines and 95 in the normal lumbar spine. We interpreted this difference to reflect that the lumbar spine is under a higher body mechanical stress than the cervical and thoracic spines. Encouraged by this fragmentary finding we prospectively extended the gamma correction value study to the entire normal bone skeleton in 18 adults of both sexes from the cranium through the axial skeleton to the appendicular bones. This chapter reports the results we attained from the ACDSee-10 gamma correction ^{99m}Tc-HDP pinhole bone scan study performed in the whole normal adult human bone skeletons to in vivo imaging-wise verify Wolff's law. Clinically, the results were unique and highly informative. Thus, we propose a graded quantitation scale of CTMF (callused trabecular microfractures): *nil* ($n = 0$), *mild* ($n = 1$–9), *moderate* ($n = 10$–29), *marked* (30–49), and *numerous* ($n \geq 50$) (Fig. 10.1).

Technically, ACDSee-10 gamma correction ^{99m}Tc-HDP pinhole bone scan can neatly image CTMF and permit to quantify it in normal adult human bones. The categorization was useful to assay physiological osteoneogenesis in the grown-up bone skeleton to imaging-wise examine Wolff's law (Wolff 1892; Monograph). The unsuppressed ^{99m}Tc-HDP uptake in CTMF precisely reflects bone metabolic state in terms of osteoneogenesis, which can be either pathological as in microfracture repair or physiological as in bone reinforcement to bear high physical stress. For information, an excellent English translation of the original Wolff's monograph entitled "Das Gesetz der Transformation der Knochen" was published by Springer-Verlag in Berlin/Heidelberg in 1986.

When processed using ACDSee-10 gamma correction the ^{99m}Tc-HDP pinhole bone scan can neatly demonstrate trabecular microfractures the smallest one of which is as small as 200 μm in size (Bahk et al. 2017, 2019). The standard of image resolution of the conventional radiograph and ^{99m}Tc-HDP pinhole bone scanning is much improved well comparing to that of conventional radiography as far as

Y.-W. Bahk, *Imaging of Trabecular Microfracture and Bone Marrow Edema and Hemorrhage*,
https://doi.org/10.1007/978-981-15-4466-8_10

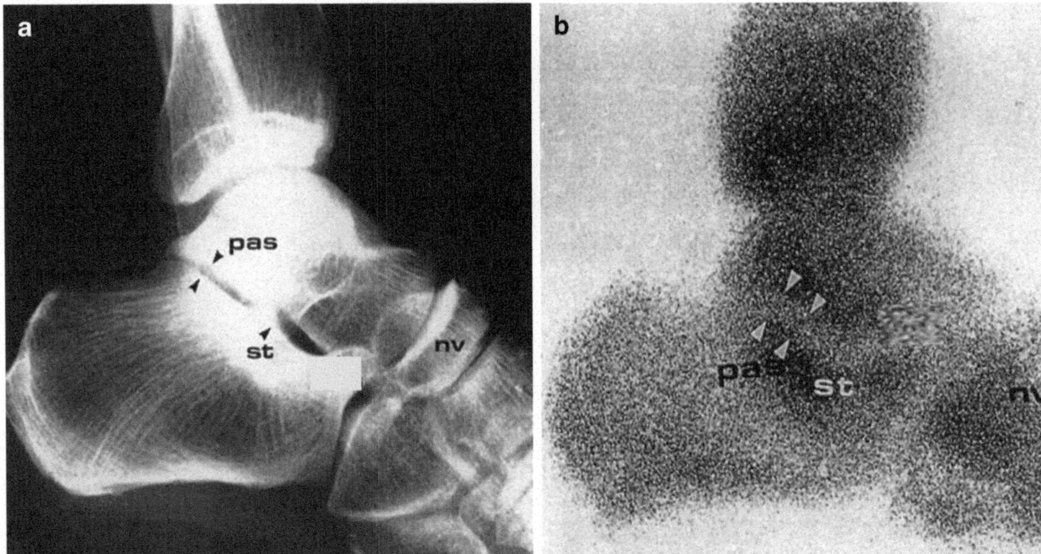

Fig. 10.1 Essentially different image presentation of conventional radiograph and ^{99m}Tc-HDP pinhole bone scan of normal adult ankle bones. (**a**) Radiograph shows the characteristic "dry" anatomic demonstration of normal trabeculae and cortical bone without any tint of bone metabolic profile. (**b**) All living bones are imaged as pinpointed tracer uptake in physiological microfractured trabeculae with variable intensity straightforwardly revealing the in vivo state of actively ongoing bone metabolism. We are convinced that such a good radiograph and ^{99m}Tc-HDP pinhole bone scan makes an ideal pair of basic bone imaging from refined anatomical and metabolic standpoints

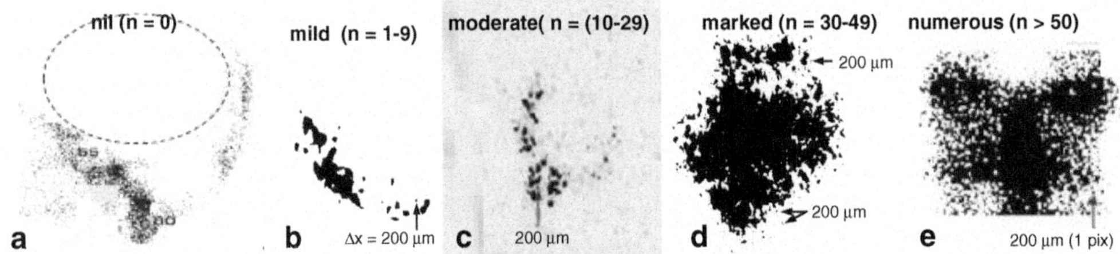

Fig. 10.2 The ^{99m}Tc-HDP pinhole bone scan processed by ACDSee-10 or ACDSee-7 gamma correction can image normal callused trabecular microfracture (CTMF) to be sorted into five categories: nil, mild, moderate, marked, and numerous. Countable CTMF is arbitrarily classified into: nil = 0, mild = 1–9, moderate = 10–29, marked = 30–49, and numerous >50. In each category, the smallest CTMF measured 200 μm in size

trabecular demonstration is concerned although the informational contents are exclusively anatomic in the former and bone metabolic in the latter (Fig. 10.2). We are convinced that such a good radiograph and refined ^{99m}Tc-HDP pinhole bone scan makes an ideal, inseparable pair of basic bone imaging dualistically from integrated, refined anatomical and metabolic standpoints.

It is considered useful that each individual bones of the entire human bone skeleton from the skull through the axis to the hand and foot bones can be neatly processed without penumbra when one uses ACDSee-10 gamma correction. For the detailed and systemic anatomical and bone metabolic information all bone skeleton attained in 18 healthy adult subjects were constructed (Fig. 10.3). Naturally, this bone metabolic atlas covers the whole bone skeleton of a human being from the skull bones, the vault, and base, through the axial spine and appendicular bones to the hands and feet including sesamoid bones. Characteristically, the whole-body gamma correction pinhole bone scanning was meticulously taken along with bone metabolism profile assessed by upgraded ACDSee-10 gamma correction. The main purpose of such an attempt is to draw a whole-body map of ^{99m}Tc-HDP pinhole bone scan metabolism in adults to examine and support the century-old Wolff's law (Fig. 10.3). We

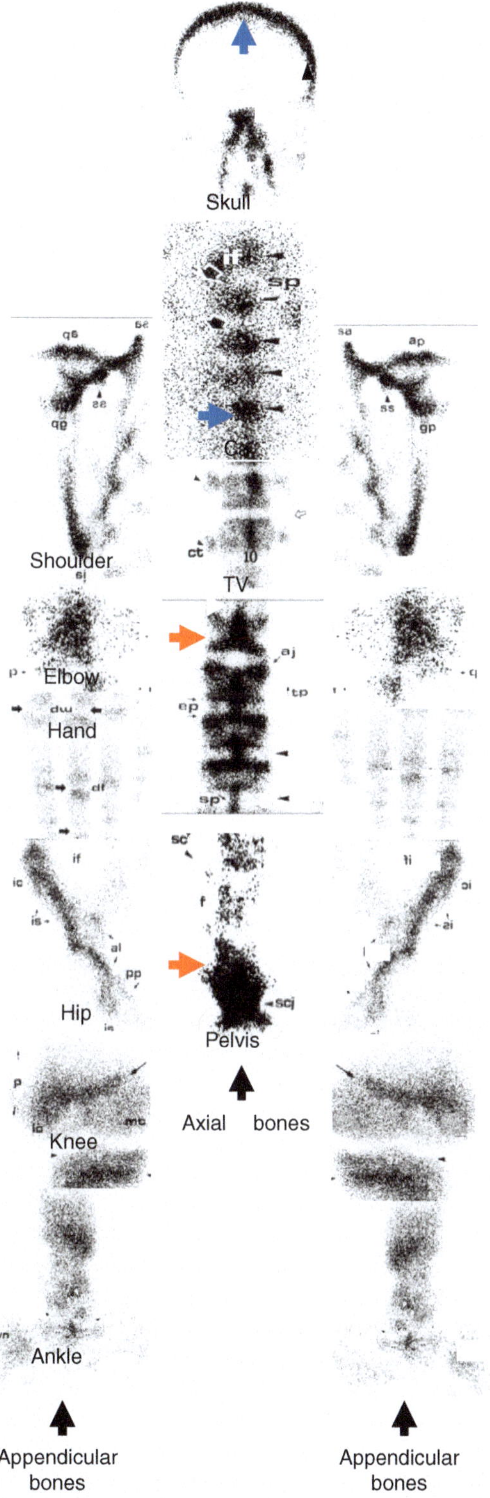

Fig. 10.3 Compounded series of ^{99m}Tc-HDP pinhole scan image processed using ACDSee-10 gamma correction of bone skeletons in 11 normal adults of both sexes show different tracer uptake patterns to support the Wolff's law. Observe that high tracer uptake particularly occurs in the axial skeleton with the highest concentration in the lumbar spine and the sacrococcygeal joint bones (red arrows). The high tracer uptake in the cranial vault and elongated spinous processes is due to sagittally accrued weak tracer uptake (blue arrows)

consider that such an attempt is worthwhile from the systemic, metabolic standpoint.

Actually, the ^{99m}Tc-HDP pinhole bone scanning of the skull, scapula, knee, and toe are purposely processed using the ACDSee-10 gamma correction to highlight the anatomical characteristics of each bone: the dome-shaped calvarial diploic bones and the irregular skull base compact bones in the skull, the flat paper-thin infraspinous cortical bone of the scapula, the stout condylar bones of the knee, and the sesamoid bones of the first metatarsal bone. The gamma correction of the skull bones showed the diploic bones of the cranial vault to be rather thickly filled with microtrabecular uptake because of the accrued accumulation of scanty CTMF which is scarce or absent in the un-overlapped thin diploic normal cranium (Fig. 10.4b). Contrary, however, the irregular skull base bones are thickly imaged presenting as a naso-ethmo-sphenoidal (NES) bone complex on the anteroposterior view (Figs. 10.4, 10.5). Being a flat compact bone the

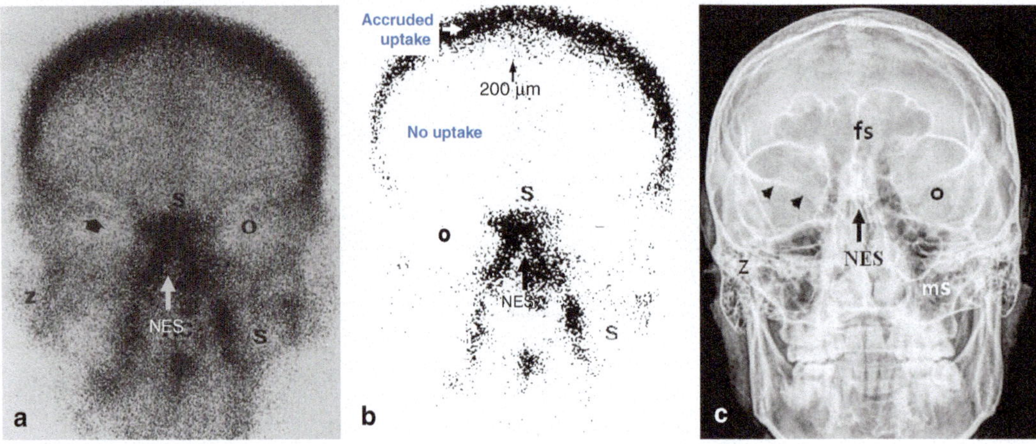

Fig. 10.4 Anteroposterior view of normal skull and facial bones. (**a**) Naive anterior ^{99m}Tc-HDP pinhole scan shows diffusely accruded increased tracer uptake in the diploic bones of the cranial vault the volume of which is sagittally accrued and the naturally complex naso-ethmo-sphenoidal (*NES*) bones in the skull base. (**b**) Gamma correction view shows accrued ^{99m}Tc-HDP uptake in the cranial vault and the skull base NES bones (arrow). Gamma correction view shows numerous 200 µm microfractures. Hollow orbits (*o*) and sinuses (*s*) are photopenic. (**c**) Radiograph identifies the diploic cranium and naso-ethmoido-sphenoidal bone complex (NES) at the skull base and the frontal and maxillary sinuses (*fs*, *ms*), orbits (*o*), and sphenoidal ridges (paired arrows). Radiograph is similar but not the same case

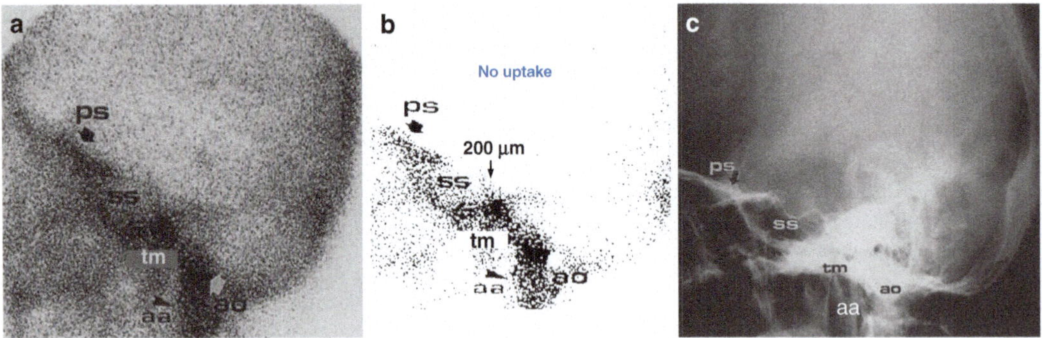

Fig. 10.5 Lateral view of normal skull base. (**a**) Naïve lateral ^{99m}Tc-HDP pinhole scan shows tracer uptake in the atlantooccipital joint (ao), temporomandibular joint (tm), sphenoid sinus (ss), and planum sphenoidale (ps). (**b**) Gamma correction view shows unsuppressed high ^{99m}Tc-HDP uptake in the skull base bones including the atlanto-occipital bone (ao), atlantoaxial temporomandibular bone (tm), sphenoid sinus (ss), and planum sphenoidale (ps). (**c**) Lateral radiograph identifies the antooccipital (ao), atlantoaxial (aa), temporomandibular (tm) bone combinations and the sphenoid sinus (ss), and planum sphenoidale (ps)

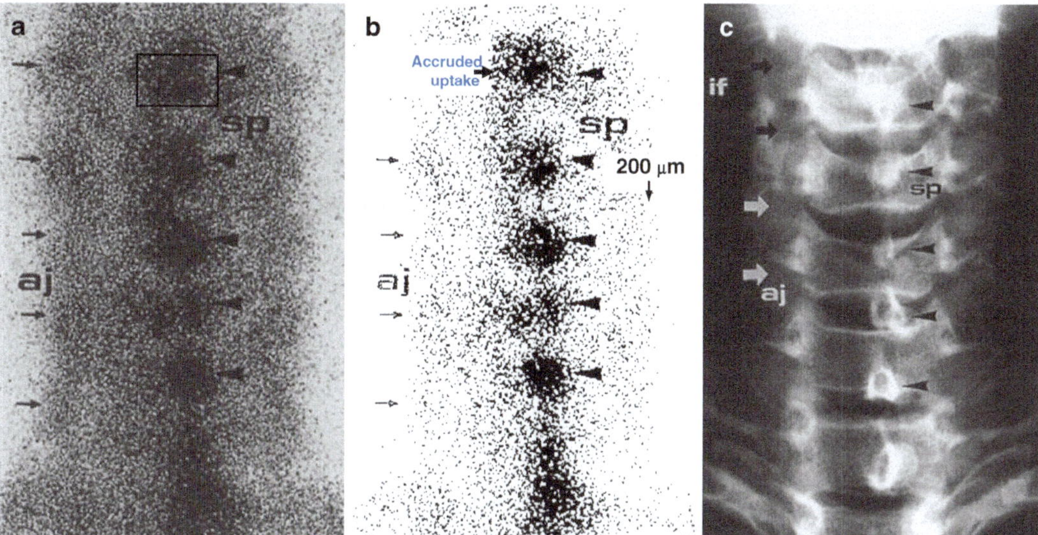

Fig. 10.6 Posterior view of normal cervical spine. (**a**) Naïve posterior ^{99m}Tc-HDP pinhole scan of the cervical spine shows accruded marked tracer uptake in the spinous processes (*sp*) and apophyseal joints (*aj*). (**b**) Gamma correction view shows accruded tracer uptake in the spinous processes (*sp*), which are sagittally imaged. (**c**) Radiograph identifies the spinous processes (*sp*), apophyseal joints (*aj*), and intervertebral foramina (*if*)

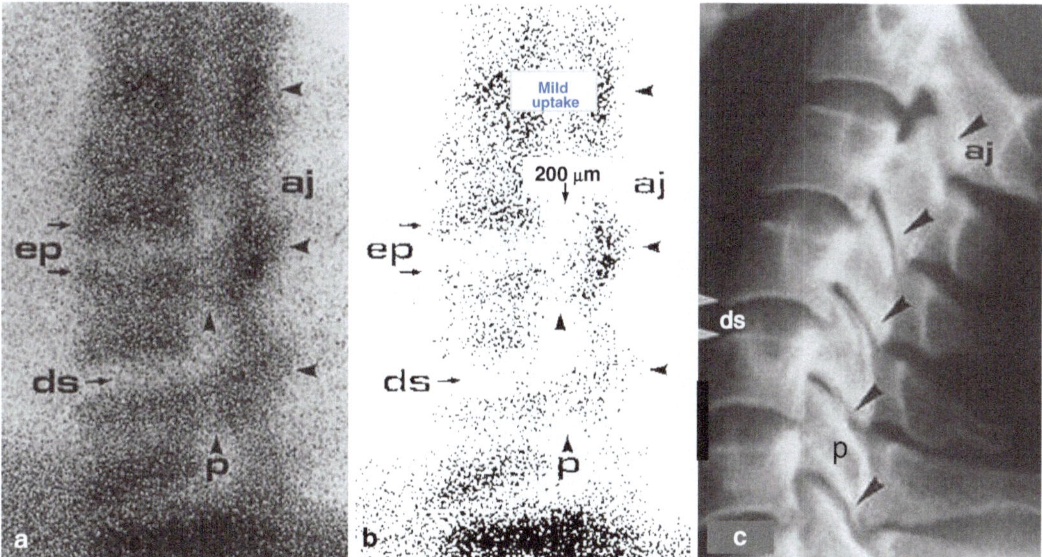

Fig. 10.7 Lateral view of normal cervical spine. (**a**) Naïve lateral ^{99m}Tc-HDP pinhole scan shows blurry moderately increased tracer uptake in the vertebral endplates (*ep*) and bodies, pedicles (*p*), and apophyseal joints (*aj*). The disk spaces show mild blurry background tracer uptake. (**b**) Gamma correction view shows numerous mild physiological pinpoint trabecular microfractures reflecting relatively mild weight bearing osteoneogenesis. (**c**) Lateral radiograph identifies the individual cervical vertebrae with endplates (white arrowheads), intervertebral disk spaces, pedicles (*p*), and apophyseal joints (*aj*; black arrowheads)

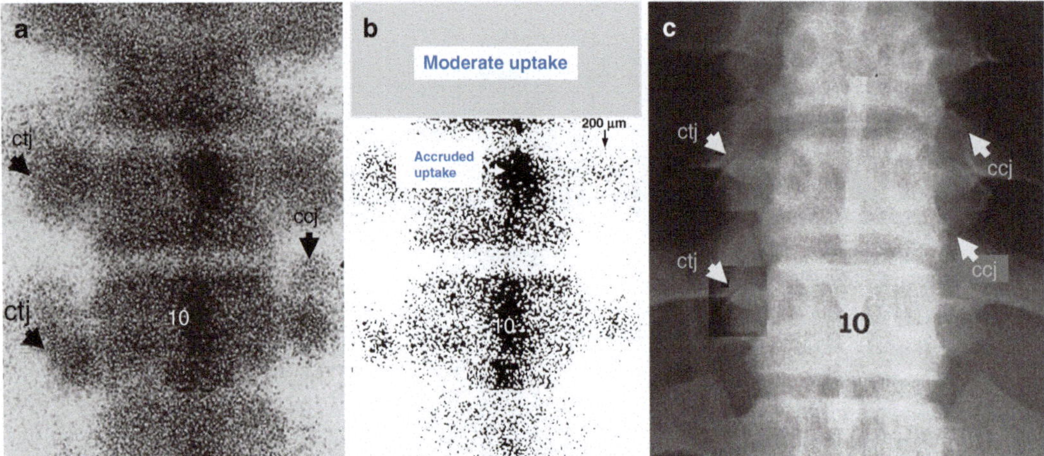

Fig. 10.8 Posteroanterior view of normal lower thoracic spine. (**a**) ^{99m}Tc-HDP pinhole scan of the lower thoracic spine shows blurry tracer uptake in the costotransverse joints (*ctj*), spinous processes, and vertebral endplates. The costocorporeal joints (*ccj*) are also demonstrated above the costotransverse joints. (**b**) Gamma correction bone scan shows numerous, physiological pinpoint trabecular microfractures presumably due to the relatively low weight bearing in the body back. (**c**) Radiograph identifies the costotransverse joint (*ctj*) formed between the transverse process and costal neck and the costocorporeal joint (*ccj*) formed between the costal head and the vertebral body

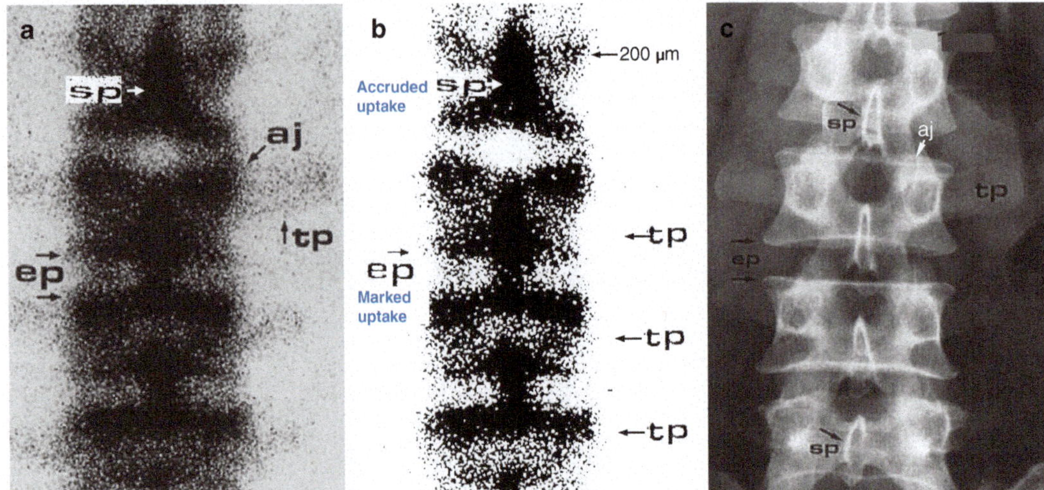

Fig. 10.9 Dorsoventral view of normal lumbar spine. (**a**) Naïve dorsal ^{99m}Tc-HDP pinhole scan of the lumbar spine shows high tracer uptake in the spinous processes (*sp*), apophyseal joints (*aj*), and vertebral endplates (*ep*) and mild uptake in the transverse process (*tp*). (**b**) Gamma correction pinhole scan shows unsuppressed marked tracer uptake in the spinous process (*sp*) and endplates (*ep*) and no uptake in the transverse processes. (**c**) Radiograph identifies the spinous processes (*sp*), apophyseal joints (*aj*), transverse process (*tp*), and vertebral endplates (*ep*). The lumbar spine shows unsuppressed marked ^{99m}Tc-HDP uptake in the endplates and spinous processes, whereas the transverse process shows no uptake reflecting that the endplates and spinous processes are under the maximum weight-bearing stress and the transverse processes are virtually free of physical stress. The difference may well be used as an advantageous tool of the imaging quantification of physical stress to bone proving Wolff's law

infraspinatus fossa of the scapula also shows the scanty microtrabeculae (Fig. 10.14) like the unoverlapped calvarial bones. In the meantime, the vulnerable knee bones consist of the femoral and tibial condyles the are functionally simple yet stout (Fig. 10.10) and finally, the great toe metatarsal bone is provided with sesamoids for articulation like the patella and the fabella in the knee. The patella is formed with thickly developed trabeculae with thin cortex. The above-mentioned difference may well be used as an advantageous tool of the imaging quantification of physical stress to bone proving Wolff's law (Wolff 1892; Frost 1994; Chen et al. 2009; Teichtahl et al.

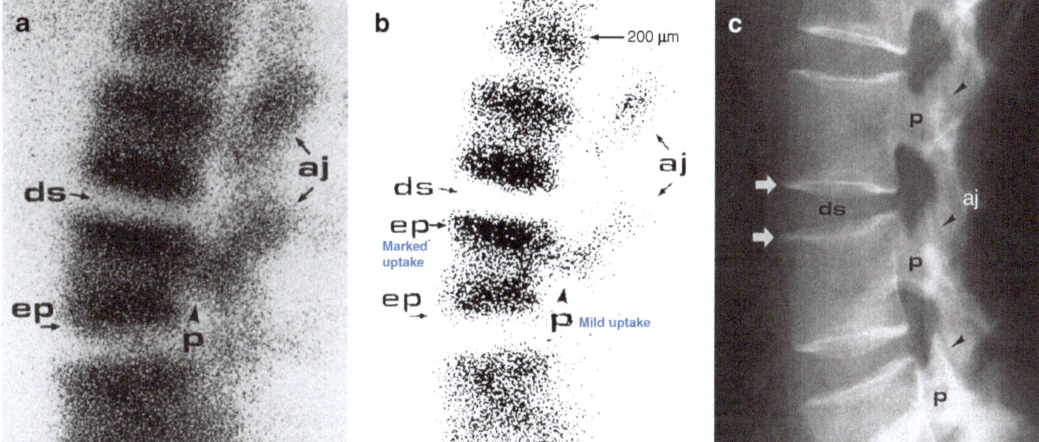

Fig. 10.10 Lateral view of normal lumbar spine. (**a**) ^{99m}Tc-HDP pinhole scan demonstrates the apophyseal joints (*aj*), disk spaces (*ds*), pedicles (*p*), and vertebral endplates (*ep*). (**b**) ACDSee-10 gamma correction pinhole scan shows unsuppressed high tracer uptake in the endplates (*ep*) and apophyseal joint (*aj*), and pedicle (*p*). (**c**) Lateral radiograph identifies the apophyseal joints (arrowheads), pedicles (*p*), disk spaces (*ds*), endplates (arrows), and apophyseal joints (arrowheads)

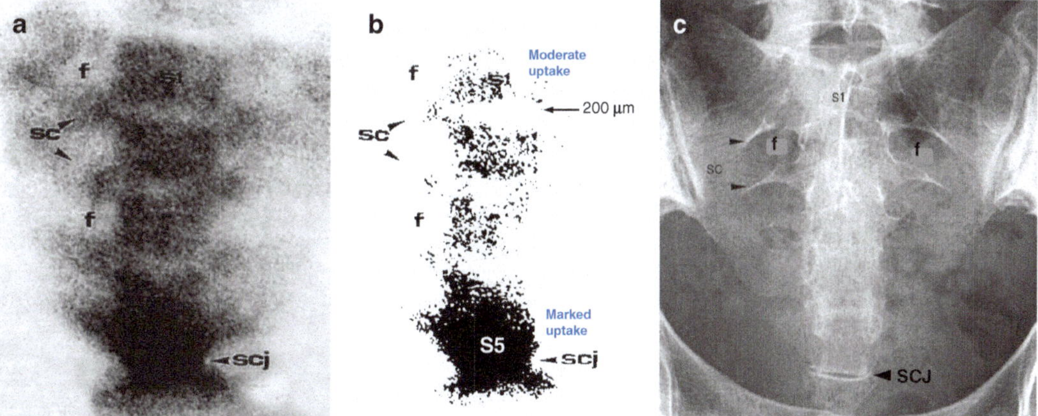

Fig. 10.11 Posterior scan and anteroposterior radiograph of normal sacrum. (**a**) Naïve ^{99m}Tc-HDP pinhole scan shows somewhat increased tracer uptake in the triangular, kite-shaped sacrum. It is the fusion of five modified vertebrae sided by photopenic foramina (*f*) and surrounded by sacral crests (*sc*). The S1 promontory is the first segment of the sacrum and termionatres at the sacrococcygeal junction (*scj*). (**b**) Gamma correction view shows the vertebrae to consist of a great number of trabecular microfractures with dense aggregation at the sacrococcygeal joint (*scj*). (**c**) Anteroposterior radiograph of a normal sacrum shows foramina delineated by the thin cortex of the sacral crests (arrowheads)

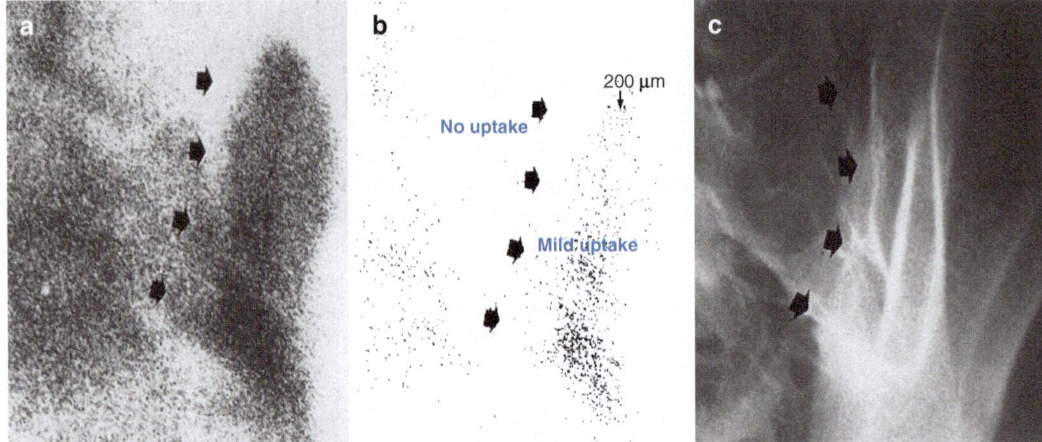

Fig. 10.12 Posterior view of normal sacroiliac joint. (**a**) Naïve ^{99m}Tc-HDP posterior pinhole scan of the left sacroiliac joint bones shows somewhat increased tracer uptake. (**b**) Gamma correction posterior tangential or butterfly pinhole scintigraph of the right sacroiliac joint separates the joint space, which is wedge-shaped in the upper compartment (arrows). Separation is incomplete in the synovial, lower compartment and complete in the ligamentous, upper compartment. The prominent tracer uptake is localized on the iliac side. (**c**) Tangential radiograph identifies the joint space between the sacrum and ilium (arrows)

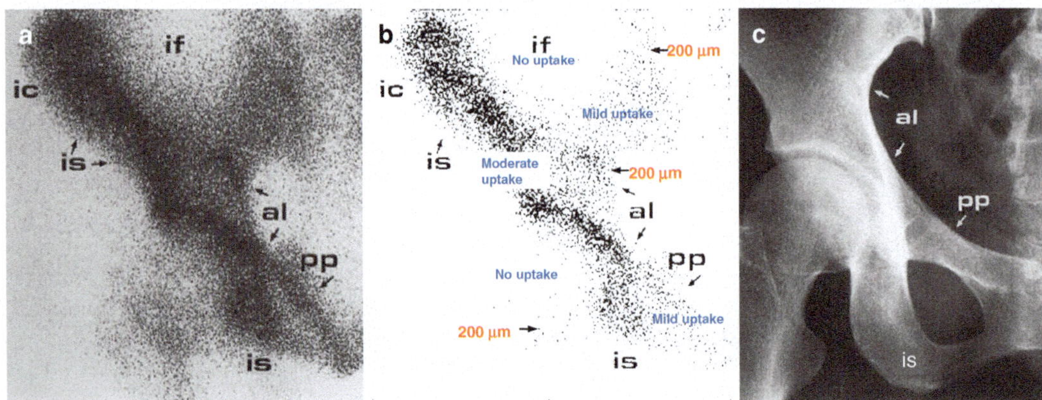

Fig. 10.13 Anterior view of normal right pelvis and hip. (**a**) Naïve anterior ^{99m}Tc-HDP pinhole scan of the right hemipelvis and hip joint reveals increased tracer uptake in the iliac crest (*ic*), iliac spine (*is*), arcuate line (*al*), pecten pubis (*pp*), ischial body (*ib*), and acetabular roof. The iliac fossa (*if*) and femoral head are shown as photopenic bones with least tracer uptake. (**b**) Gamma correction view characteristically shows modest tracer uptake in the iliac crest and spine and acetabular fossa. Observe the smallest microfracture to measure 200 μm in size. (**c**) Anteroposterior radiograph identifies the arcuate line (*al*), pecten pubis (*pp*), ischium (*is*), and pubic body as well as the acetabular fossa

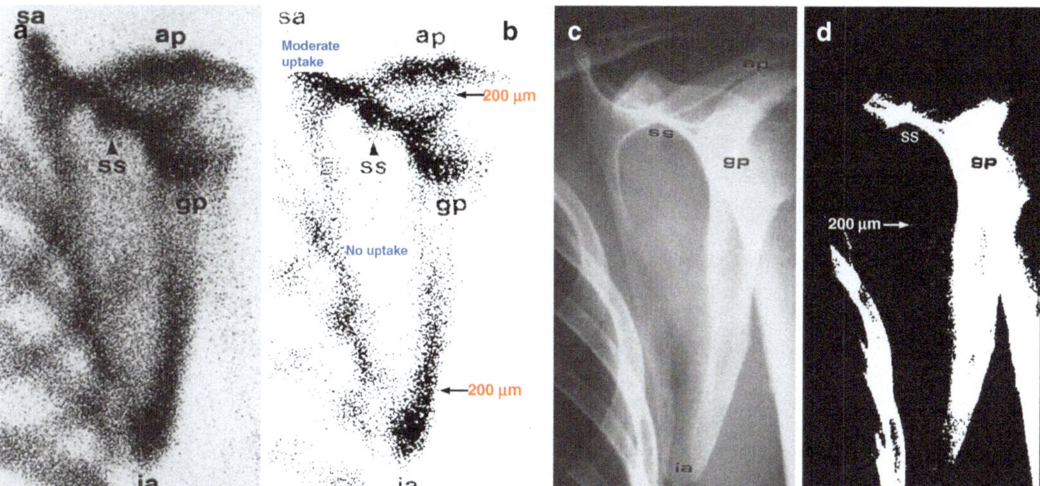

Fig. 10.14 Normal semilateral view of the scapula showing the infraspinatus fossa to consist of typical compact bone. (**a**) Semilateral pinhole scan of the left scapula shows intense tracer uptake in the acromion process (*ap*), spina scapularis (*ss*), glenoid process (*gp*), and the superior and inferior angles (*sa* and *ia*). (**b**) Gamma correction suppresses tracer uptake in the compact infraspinous fossa bone with very scanty physiological microfractures. (**c**) Naïve radiograph identifies the spina scapularis (*ss*), superior (*sa*) and inferior scapular angles (*fa*), acromion (*ap*), and glenoid processes (*gp*). (**d**) Gamma correction radiograph shows the infraspinous fossa to contain scanty physiological callused trabecular microfractures which measure 200 µm in size

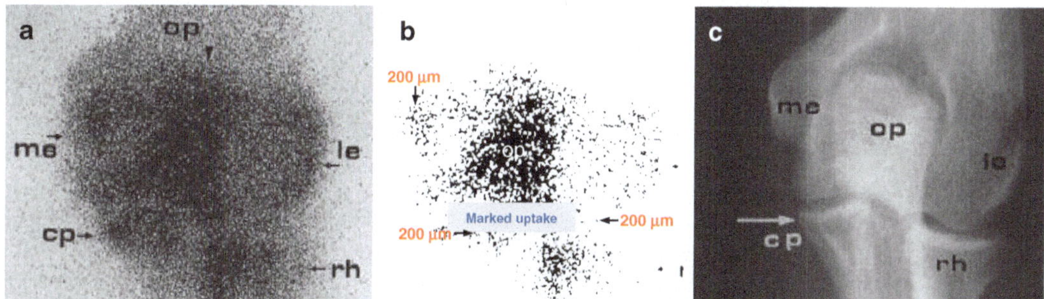

Fig. 10.15 Ventrodorsal views of normal elbow. (**a**) Naïve ^{99m}Tc-HDP anterior pinhole scan shows blurry tracer uptake in the olecranon process (*op*), medial and lateral epicondyles (*me*, *le*), coronoid process (*cp*), and radial head (*rh*). (**b**) Gamma correction shows highlighted aggregation of mottled and pinpointed tracer uptake with the smallest ones measuring 200 µm in size. (**c**) Radiograph identifies the olecranon process (*op*), medial and lateral epicondyles (*me*, *le*), coronoid process (*cp*), and radial head (*rh*)

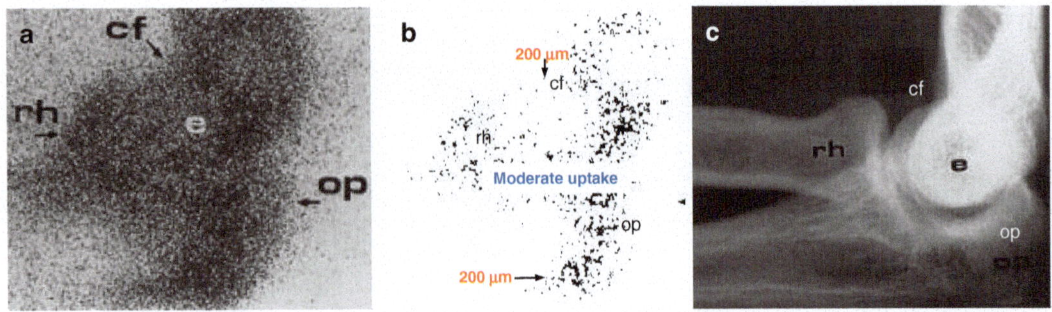

Fig. 10.16 Lateral views of normal elbow. (**a**) Naïve lateral pinhole scan shows the coronoid fossa (*cf*), radial head (*rh*), epicondyles (*e*), and olecranon process (*op*). (**b**) Gamma correction view shows irregular mottled and pinpointed highlighted tracer uptake with the smallest measuring 200 µm in size. (**c**) Radiograph identifies the coronoid fossa (*cf*), radial head (*rh*), epicondyles (*e*), and olecranon process (*op*)

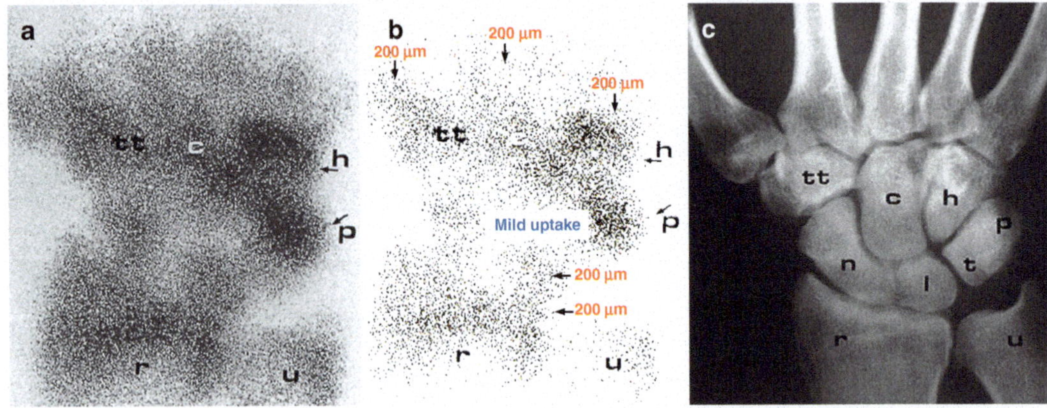

Fig. 10.17 Dorsoventral view of the normal right wrist. (**a**) Naïve dorsal ^{99m}Tc-HDP pinhole scan of the right wrist shows minimal increased tracer uptake in the distal ends of the radius (*r*) and ulna (*u*), and the four proximal carpal bones: the navicular (*n*), lunate (*l*), triquetral (*t*), and pisiform (*p*). (**b**) Gamma correction pinhole scan shows suppression of blurry racer uptake highlighting trabecular microfractures in the distal radius (*r*) and ulna (*u*) and navicular (*n*), lunate (*l*), triquetral (*t*), pisiform (*p*), trapezoid and trapezium (*tt*), capitatum (*c*), and hamatum (*h*) bones. (**c**) Radiograph identifies the radius (*r*) and ulna (*u*) as well as eight carpal bones including the navicular (*n*), lunate (*l*), triquetral (*t*), and pisiform (*p*)

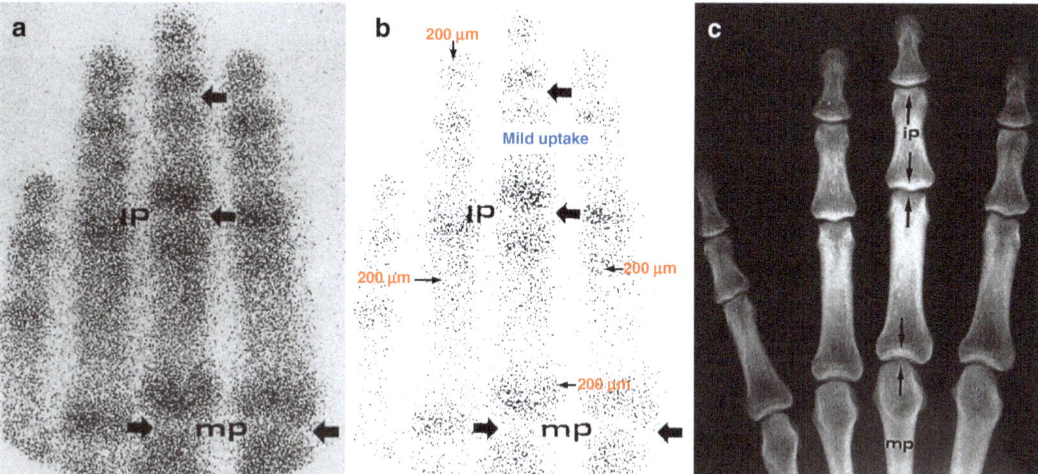

Fig. 10.18 Dorsoventral view of normal left hand fingers. (**a**) Naïve ^{99m}Tc-HDP pinhole scan shows the metacarpophalangeal (*mp*) and interphalangeal joints (*ip*). Tracer accumulates mainly in the bases and heads of the phalanges showing joints (arrows). (**b**) Gamma correction view suppresses blurry tracer uptake highlighting numerous trabecular microfractures and interphalangeal joints. (**c**) Dorsoventral radiograph identifies the metacarpophalangeal (*mp*) and interphalangeal joints (*ip*). The thumb is not included because of the space

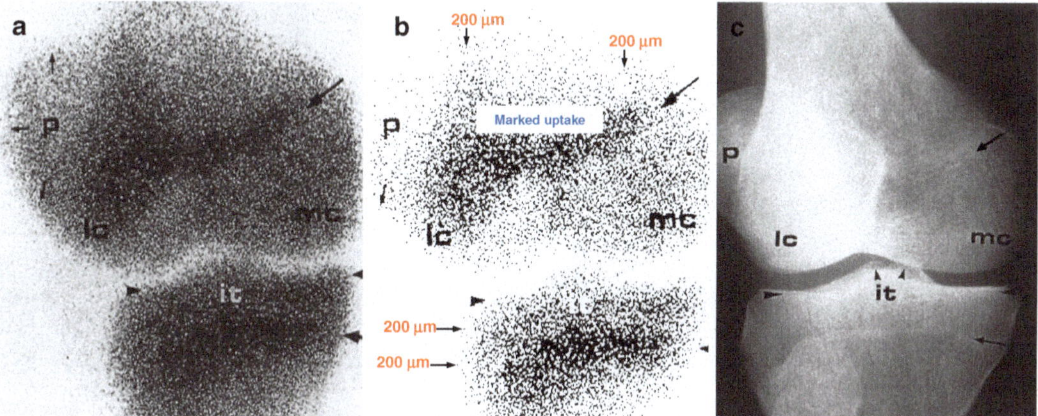

Fig. 10.19 Anteroposterior view of the right knee. (**a**) Anterior pinhole scan of demonstrates increased tracer uptake in the medial and lateral femoral condyles (*mc*, *lc*), patella (*p*), intercondylar tubercles of the tibia (*it*), and tibial plateaus (arrowheads). The closed physeal lines in the distal femur and proximal tibia are indicated by blurry transverse tracer uptake (large arrows). (**b**) Gamma correction view shows numerous trabecular microfractures. (**c**) Anteroposterior radiograph identifies the medial and lateral femoral condyles (*mc*, *lc*), tibial intercondylar tubercles (*it*), tibial plateau (horizontal arrowheads), and patella (*p*). The closed physeal lines are faintly visible in the distal femur and proximal tibia (arrows)

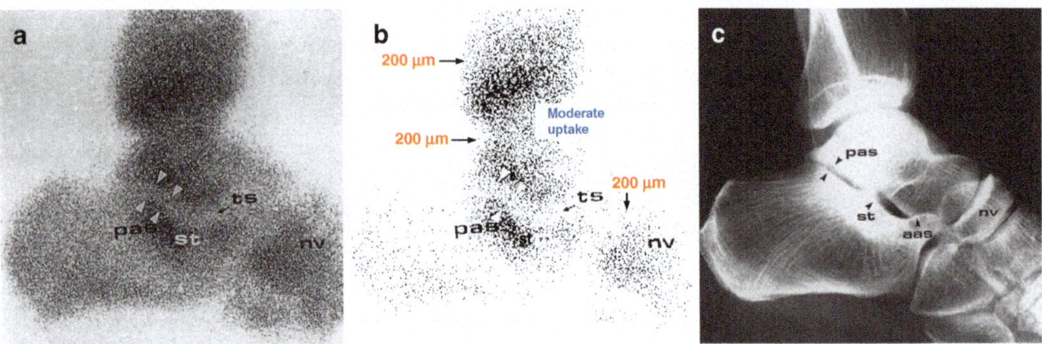

Fig. 10.20 Mediolateral views of the left ankle. (**a**) Naïve mediolateral ^{99m}Tc-HDP pinhole scan of the hindfoot shows minimally increased tracer uptake in the posterior articular surfaces of the talus and calcaneus (*pas*, arrowheads), sustentaculum tali (*st*), and tarsal sinus (*ts*). The navicular bone (*nv*) is also visualized. (**b**) Gamma correction view highlights numerous caluswed trabecular microfractures. (**c**) Mediolateral radiograph identifies the posterior articular surfaces of the talus and calcaneus (*pas*, arrowheads), the sustentaculum tali (*st*), and the anterior articular surface of the calcaneus (*aas*). The tarsal sinus (*ts*) is shown as a bone-free slit between the talus and calcaneus

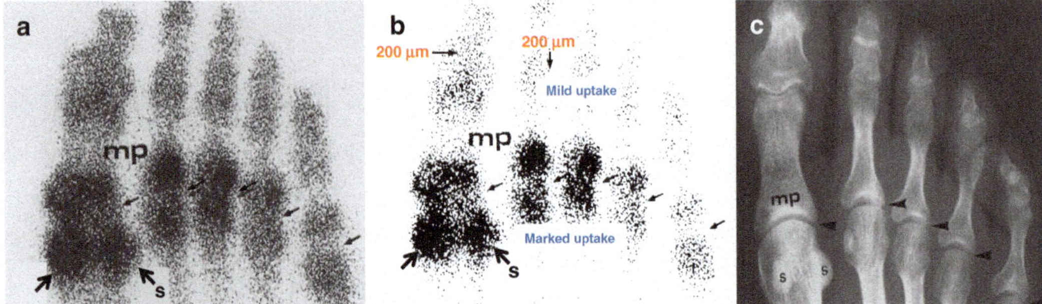

Fig. 10.21 Normal dorsoplanter right forefoot. (**a**) Naïve ^{99m}Tc-HDP pinhole scan shows nonspecific tracer uptake in metatarsophalangeal joint bones of five toes (*mp*, arrows). Sesamoids show high physiological tracer uptake due to articulation (arrows). (**b**) Gamma correction view shows numerous physiological 200-µm microfractures in ceaselessly walking feet. (**c**) Naïve radiograph shows metatarsophalangeal joints (*mp*, arrowheads) and sesamoid bones (*s*)

2015; Alexander and Elma 2016; and Dorland's Illustrated Medical Dictionary 32nd ed. Elsevier). The figures, not individually presented in this discussion, were necessarily included to make up the whole 99mTc-HDP pinhole scan atlas.

Indeed, this ACDsee-10 gamma correction ^{99m}Tc-HDP pinhole bone scan atlas of the entire bone skeleton of adult Korean is elaborated for the demonstration of the uniqueness and usefulness of enhanced gamma correction for the systematic pinhole-bone-scan anatomy and bone metabolism assessment. Naturally, our atlas includes the skull, axial bones, and all appendicular bones including the fingers and toes. It is not only bone anatomico-metabolically informative but also a useful in vivo imaging evidence to support classic Wolff's law. This method can also be used as a handy in vivo imaging tool of the anatomico-metabolical assay of the human adult bone skeleton, individually and systematically.

References

Alexander SA, Elma ST. The birth of a new scientific field – biomechanics of the skeleton. Julius Wolff and his work "Das Gesetz der Transformation der Knochen.". Hist Med. 2016;3:372–6. https://doi.org/10.17720/2409-5834.v.4.2016.36q.

Bahk YW, Hwang SH, Lee UY, et al. Morphobiochemical diagnosis of acute trabecular microfractures using gamma correction Tc-99m HDP pinhole bone scan with histopathological verification. Medicine. 2017;96(45):e8419.

Bahk YW, Kim EE, Chung YA, et al. Precise differential diagnosis of acute bone marrow edema and hemorrhage and trabecular microfractures using naïve and gamma correction pinhole bone scans. J Int Med Res. 2019; https://doi.org/10.1177/0300060518819910.

Chen JH, Chao L, Lictan Y, et al. Boning upon Wolff's law: mechanical regulation of the cells that make and maintain bone. J Biomech. 2009; https://doi.org/10.1016/j.jbiomech.

Dorland. Dorland's illustrated medical dictionary. 32nd ed. Philadelphia: Elsevier Saunders; 2012. p. 1011.

Frost HM. Wolff's law and bone's structural adaptations to mechanical usage: an overview for clinicians. Angle Orthod. 1994;64(3):175–88.

Teichtahl A, Wluka A, Wijthilake P. Wolff's law in action: a mechanism for early knee osteoarthritis. Arthritis Res Ther. 2015; https://doi.org/10.1185/s13075-015-0738-7.

Wolff J. Ueber die innere Architectur der Knochen und ihre Beteutung für die Frage vom Knochenwachsthum. In: Das Gesetz der Transformation von Knochen. This was published as a monograph in Berlin by Verlag von August Hirschwald; 1892.

11 ACDSee-10 Gamma Correction MRI for Neat Imaging and Magnifying Lens Measurement of Callused Trabecular Microfracture

The excelled usefulness of gamma correction ^{99m}Tc-HDP pinhole bone scan for the imaging and diagnosis of callused trabecular microfracture (CTMF) has been well demonstrated and discussed. Now in succession, the same principle of gamma correction of ACDSee-10 version is practically considered to be worthy of importing to magnetic resonance imaging (MRI) to make an in vivo demonstration of CTMF, which occurs in most bone diseases and also in normal bones. Special MRI techniques such as proton spectroscopy and multiparametry can show nearly all kinds of somatic tissues and organs, but apparently excepting trabecular microfracture. Recently, we became to realize that ACDSee-10 gamma correction MRI can visualize and quantitate CTMF (Vide Chap. 13). The aims of this study on ACDSee-10 gamma correction MRI are twofold: first is an extended application of gamma correction to MRI for precise, graphic diagnosis of CTMF by avoiding penumbra and second is to develop handy quantitation method in terms of the number of injured pixel simply using a magnifying lens. Technically, we imaged microfractures by seriated naive and ACDSee-10 gamma correction T2 weighted MRI in *nine* consecutive cases. The clinical materials consisted of the bones of the shoulder girdle, hip, knee, ankle, and foot. The usefulness of ACDSee-10 gamma correction MRI diagnosis was verified in each case by the corroboratory trabecular microfracture findings of foregone ACDSee-10 ^{99m}Tc-HDP *pinhole bone scan* and surgical specimen as well as H&E stain. Results were that the bright MR signal intensity of microfracture was distinctly highlighted and precisely measured by the direct counting of the number of injured pixel using a magnifying optic lens. *The injured micrometric* pixel was characteristically presented as bright signal intensity against dark background matrix on ACDSee-10 gamma correction MRI, while it was conversely presented as dark microscopic ^{99m}Tc-HDP uptake against bright matrix on ACDSee 10 gamma correction pinhole bone scan. The latter was used to validate the former. The smallest size of the unit pixel shown in our computer screen was 200 μm in the *x*-axis of coordinate. ACDSee-10 gamma correction MRI demonstrated as many as *15* single-pixel CTMF in nine cases, but ACDSee 10 gamma correction pinhole bone scan showed only *five* single-pixel CTMF and such a difference was theoretically presumed to be due to high sensitivity of MRI. For information, the diagonal of computer monitor we used was 24 inches and screen resolution was 1920 × 1080, Samsung LS23C340, Seoul, South Korea.

Generally, the injured integuments and internal organ tissues in human body heal by fibrous scar, but exceptionally trabecular microfracture is cured by osteoneogenesis in the form of callus and endosteal rimming. As well known, the callus is unorganized meshwork of woven bone developed on the fibrin clot, which will be

Y.-W. Bahk, *Imaging of Trabecular Microfracture and Bone Marrow Edema and Hemorrhage*,
https://doi.org/10.1007/978-981-15-4466-8_11

ultimately replaced by adult bone (Dorland 2012). It is formed to heal trabecular microfracture in traumatized bone (Vernon-Roberts and Pirie 1973; Mandalia and Henson 2008), osteoporosis (Frost 1973), aseptic osteonecrosis (McFarland and Frost 1961), inflammatory, infective, metabolic, and neoplastic diseases of bone (Bahk 2017), laborious work and sports stresses, and even in normal daily physical activities (Fazzarali 1993). Clinically, the mild osteoneogenesis in CTMF can be physiological but when systemic it may become an important health and economic problems, especially in highly aged subjects (Tassani and Matsopoulos 2013). Until now, CTMF was assessed using ACDSee gamma correction limitedly in ^{99m}Tc-HDP pinhole bone scan (Bahk et al. 2016, 2017) and gamma correction was not used in MRI. Lately, we became to learn that ACDSee-10 retrieved from https://www.altools.co.kr (ALSee. 2018 December) can be usefully imported to MRI (Fig.11.1a, b) not only to demonstrate microfracture but also to precisely quantify it using an ordinary magnifying lens (Fig. 11.1e). Thus, we applied it to standard 1.5-T MRI and results thereby attained were visually analyzed and validated using the foregoing ACDSee-10 gamma-corrected ^{99m}Tc-HDP pinhole bone scan (Fig. 11.1d), and histological studies using (1) surgical specimen analysis (Fig.11.1f), (2) surgical surface microscopy (Fig. 11.1g), and (3) H&E stain (Fig. 11.1h).

The MRI reinforced with proton MR spectroscopy is widely used in the fine anatomical study of bone diseases (Fayad et al. 2012) and the multiparametric evaluation to diagnose musculoskeletal tumors (Partovi et al. 2015), but not for the diagnosis of osteoneogenesis in CTMF. Recently, the ACDSee-10 gamma correction was imported to MRI finding that it could ideally visualize trabecular microfracture along with bone metabolic information in terms of bright signal intensity change (Fig. 11.1a,b). Methodologically, CTMF was distinctly highlighted by the suppression of edema and hemorrhage and the number of so highlighted trabeculae varied from single and a

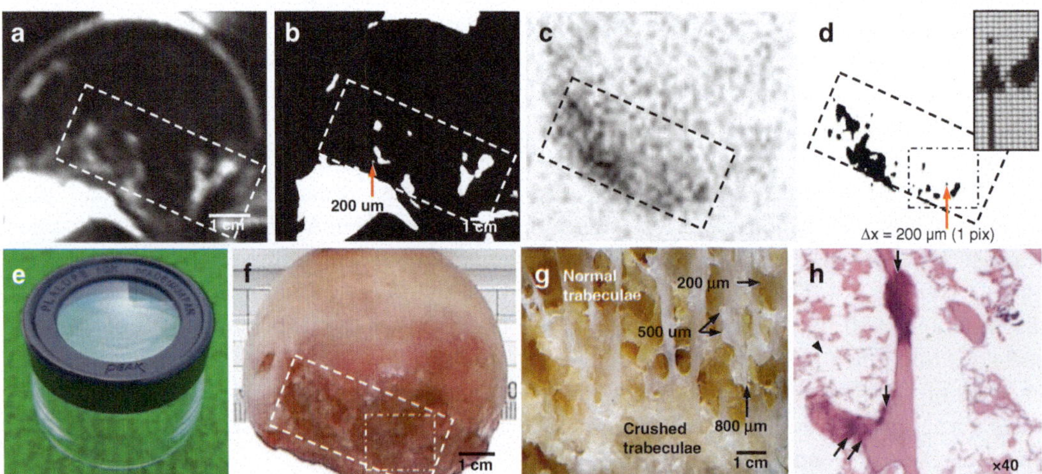

Fig. 11.1 ACDSee-10 gamma correction MRI demonstration and quantitation of 200-µm callused trabecular microfracture in the right femoral neck presented as bright signal intensity on gamma correction MRI in a 72-year-old female. (**a**) Naïve coronal T2 WT MR image of fractured right femoral neck shows nonspecific blurry tracer uptake (*frame*). (**b**) Gamma correction MR image highlights 200-µm microcallus. (**c**) Naïve ^{99m}Tc-HDP pinhole bone scan shows blurry tracer uptake (*frame*). (**d**) ACDSee-10 gamma correction pinhole bone scan shows micro- and macrotrabecular fractures with the smallest one measuring 200 µm in size. Inset is the close-up view of microcallus taken by built-in camera in cell phone. (**e**) Ten-fold magnifying lens. (**f**) Surgically removed femoral head and neck. Smaller frame denotes ROI. (**g**) Surface microscope shows the demonstration of seed-pearly trabecular mcrofractures with the smallest one measuring 200 um in size. (**h**) H&E stain shows characteristic base stained microfractures and fat cells and edema and hemorrhage

few to many and more often than not even to numerous. Additionally, ACDSee-10 gamma correction demonstration of the smallest 200 μm pixel can be easily achieved because the injured pixel is neatly highlighted as a microspot. The microspot was bright against the dark matrix signal intensity of MR image as shown in Fig. 11.1a, b, whereas it is contrarily highlighted as dark tracer uptake against bright matrix on gamma correction pinhole bone scan as shown in Fig. 11.1d. Note that the smallest microfracture involves one single pixel which measures 200 μm in size (Fig. 11.1d inset).

Systematically analyzed CTMF demonstrated in *nine* cases of seriated naïve and ACDSee-10 enhanced gamma correction T2 weighted FS MRI in this study. The diagnosis was confirmed in each case based on the characteristic CTMF shown on both ACDSee-10 pinhole bone scan and H&E stain (Fig. 11.1d, g, h) (Bahk et al. 2016, 2017). Study materials included six males and three females and their ages ranged from 15 to 71 years with the average being 38.2 years. The microfracture involved the bones of the shoulder girdle (2 cases), knee (4 cases), ankle (2 cases), and foot ($n = 1$). This imaging study was approved by the Institutional Review Board. What we used were only MRI and bone scan without any physical participation of patients wavering consent. However, one patient agreed and signed informed consent for the use of his operated femoral head specimen.

For this investigation, the most common 1.5-tesla Avanto model of MRI and E-cam Signature pinhole gamma camera system of Siemens, Knoxville, ILL, USA was used. MR image and pinhole bone scan were processed in succession by ACDSee-10 gamma correction photo editor. The number of pixel(s) of microcallus shown by ACDSee-10 gamma correction MRI and pinhole bone scan ranged from single to multiple, and unit pixel was 200 μm or 0.2 mm in size, which was easily counted by a tenfold magnifying lens (Fig. 11.1e). Naïve T2 weighted FS MR image and naïve ^{99m}Tc-HDP pinhole scan were blurry at the first looking because of edema and hemorrhage, but the blur was suppressed by ACDSee-10 gamma correction neatly highlighting microfracture both in MRI image and in pinhole bone scan (Fig. 11.1b, d). We used ACDSee-7 gamma correction in our earlier studies (Bahk et al. 2016, 2017), but it was recently changed to ACDSee-10 version, which can more sharply and sensitively image microfractures. Advantageously enough, upgraded ACDSee-10 gamma correction visualized neatly defined CTMF by eliminating penumbra and could additionally image an increased number of trabecular microinjuries because of enhanced imaging sensitivity. The upgraded gamma correction effects of ACDS-10 version compared to SCDSee 7 was tested and confirmed in two different ways; the one is by performing ^{99m}Tc-HDP pinhole bone scan test (Fig. 11.2 top panel) and the other one is performing MRI test of tibial tuberosity contusion (Fig. 11.2 bottom panel). This comparison study confirmed that the upgraded version of ACDSee-10 is by far superior to the version 7.

In regard to methodology, it is here to be remarked again that the micrometric size of CTMF in this study derived from < - > which measures 1 mm in length consisting of 5 pixels in the x-axis on the computer screen. The result attained was that the smallest unit pixel is 200 μm in size. Based on this pixel scale, we measured the callused microfracture size using a magnifying lens (Figs. 11.1e, g). Computer monitor used was 24-inches in the diagonal and screen resolution was 1920 × 1080 (LG 24MP58VG, Seoul, Korea). Screen resolution was important as the size and number of pixel shown on it are thereon closely dependent. Actually, we took naïve coronal T2 weighted FS MR image (Fig. 11.1a) and processed it using ACDSee-10 to highlight CTMF (Fig.11.1b). So, enhanced gamma correction MR image visualized microcalluses with bright signal intensity against dark matrix (Fig. 11.1b). The sequential procedures of image processing of ACDSee-10 are to be described here in a little more detail. The naïve MR image is imported to ACDSee-10, and the "filter" in the top menu bar is selected. Then, select the "Exposure/Lighting" and "Exposure" again. There are three sliding bars to control: (1) Exposure, (2) Contrast, and (3) Fill Light. The default values in the control bar are all set to

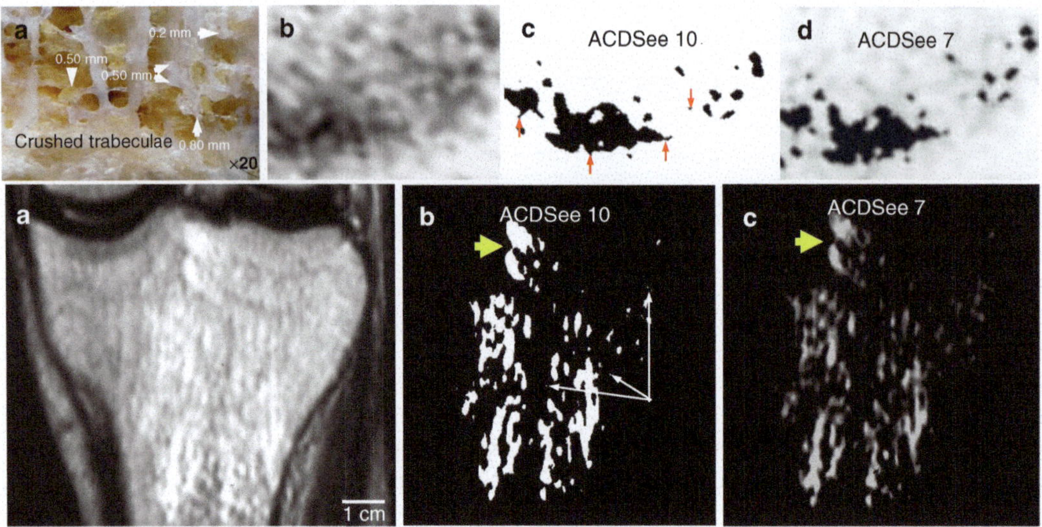

Fig. 11.2 Improved definition and high sensitivity of ACDSee-10 gamma correction image than ACDSee-7 gamma correction image in surgically removed femoral head in a 72-year-old female patient and obvious difference of ACDSee 10 and ACDSee 7 gamma correction views of callused trabecular fractures in another 78-year-old male patient. **Top panel case:** (**a**) Microscopy of femoral neck shows microfractures. (**b**) Naïve ^{99m}Tc-HDP pinhole scan shows nonspecific blurry tracer uptake (**c**) ACDSee-10 gamma correction shows sharply defined microfractures (*arrows*). Smaller calluses are imaged due to increased sensitivity. (**d**) ACDSee-7 gamma correction pinhole scan shows fractures with penumbra. **Bottom panel case:** (**a**) Naïve T2 WT FS coronal MR image shows numerous blurry bright signal intensities. (**b**) ACDSee-10 correction shows several micrometric microcalluses (*arrows*). (**c**) ACDSee-7 gamma correction MR image is blurry due to penumbra (*arrow*). Observe that upgraded gamma correction can far more neatly image 200-μm microcalluses (*small arrows*) which are unseen and undiagnosed by ACDSee-7 gamma correction

zeros. In our study, exposure and contrast were particularly enhanced in both MRI and ^{99m}Tc-HDP pinhole scan presented in the black-and-white mode. It is considered that the control of "exposure" provides the dynamic range of luminance in which we are interested and the control of contrast may amplify the perception of luminance in our eyes. After editing the image to optimally visualize the microcallus, the final image is saved with another new name. Further details can be found in Cambridge in Color).

Thus, the ACDSee-10 enhanced gamma correction was successfully imported to MRI to individually image CTMF and the findings thereby attained were validated using ACDSee-10 gamma correction pinhole bone scan and H&E stain in patients (Bahk et al. 2017). Basically, naïve pinhole bone scan was taken using Siemens E-cam signature, Knoxville, ILL, USA. It was equipped with a 4-mm pinhole collimator. The scan factors were 925–1110 MBq (25–30 mCi) ^{99m}Tc-HDP, 7-min scan time, and 12-cm pinhole-aperture-to-object distance to enough encompass all bones of the four major joints of the shoulder girdle, hip, knee, and ankle. Practically, gamma correction was performed by clicking the toolbars as described in naïve and gamma correction MR imaging and the size of callus was directly measured using a 10× magnifying lens. For technical information, ACDSee-10 gamma correction of trabecular microfracture in MRI was achieved by decreasing gamma value to, for example, below 35 from 50 (default value) and contrarily by increasing gamma value up to 95 in pinhole bone scan.

As earlier mentioned, a pixel was determined to be positively injured only when it is presented with enough brightness on ACDSee-10 enhanced MRI and enough darkness on the gamma correction pinhole scan. The defective or faint presentation was regarded as not positive. Actually, the digitalized image of CTMF as shown on the

ACDSee-10 enhanced MR image was counted in terms of pixel. To reiterate the < - > was the basic scale of pixel size that consists of five 0.2-mm pixels. The number of injured pixels could be counted using a 10× magnifying optic lens. The computer monitor used was 24 inches in diagonal and screen resolution was 1920 × 1080 (Samsung LS23C340. Seoul, Korea). To be exact one 0.2-mm pixel was the smallest unit of microfracture in this study.

On the one hand, the use of the findings of gamma correction of ACDSee-10 pinhole bone scan could confirm and validate CTMF as it is assessed in terms of pixel involvement using an ordinary 10x magnifying optic lens (Fig. 11.1h) (Bahk et al. 2016, 2017). On the one hand the number of injured pixel was counted in the *x*- and/or *y*-axis of coordinate and the counting was converted to micron. When injured pixel was single the size was 200 μm and multiple the sizes varied from 0.4 mm, 0.6 mm, and so forth. On the other hand, ACDSee-10 enhanced gamma correction was performed to radiobiochemically distinguish unfixed ^{99m}Tc-HDP uptake from fixed uptake. Characteristically, the unfixed low tracer uptake was neatly suppressed by gamma correction, but fixed high uptake was not. It is recommended that naïve ^{99m}Tc-HDP pinhole bone scan is to be processed using ACDSee-10 to precisely and more sensitively visualize CTMF without penumbra in ^{99m}Tc-HDP pinhole bone scan (Fig. 11.2 top panel) and also in MRI (Fig. 11.2 bottom panel).

Technically the gamma value in bone scan was increased up to 95 so that the unfixed low tracer uptake in edema and hemorrhage were suppressed by clicking the toolbars in the following sequence (Jung et al. 2016): exposure and image-brightness control were done by increasing gamma value up to 95 starting from 50 (the default value in Photo Editor) and done and save the final image with another new name. The use of original naïve digital information and communications in medicine (DICOM) scan without image modification was required.

In order to confirm and validate the accuracy of 10× magnifying lens measurement, we meticulously compared the values of measurement of the individual microcalluses formed in trabecular microfractures using both magnifying lens measurements and computed pixel calculation (Fig. 11.3). Corroborative assessment of both methods showed an excellent match.

11.1 General Considerations

We prospectively assessed the clinical usefulness of the diagnosis of ACDSee-10 gamma correction T2 weighted FS MRI of actively forming CTMF in *nine* consecutive cases. Objects included the bones of the shoulder girdle, hip, knee, ankle, and foot. For validation ACDSee-10 gamma correction ^{99m}Tc-HDP pinhole bone scan and H&E stain were used. In each case, the diagnosis CTMF was confirmed by typical gamma

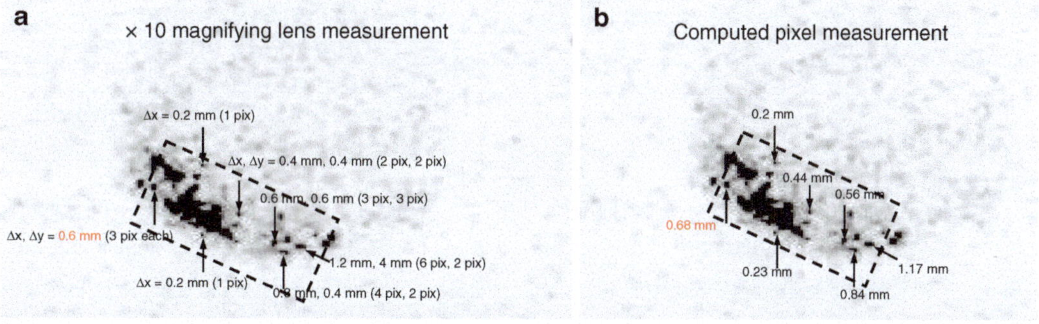

Fig. 11.3 The equalityof 10× magnifying lens measurement (n = 7) and computed pixel measurement (n = 7) of callused trabecular microfracture size. All measurements were equal except for the one at the most left laterally located one (red colored). The difference was 0.6 mm and 0.68 mm

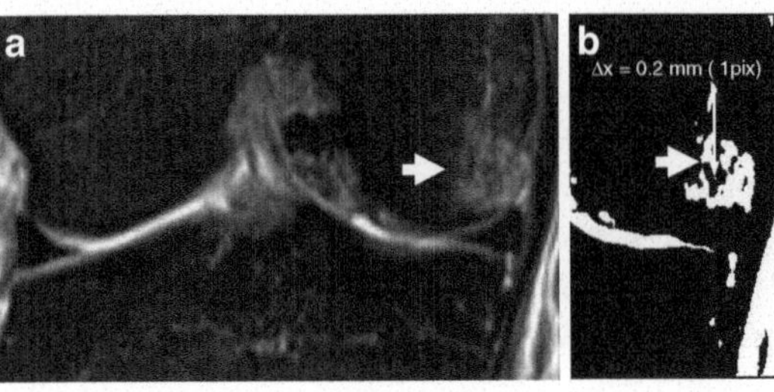

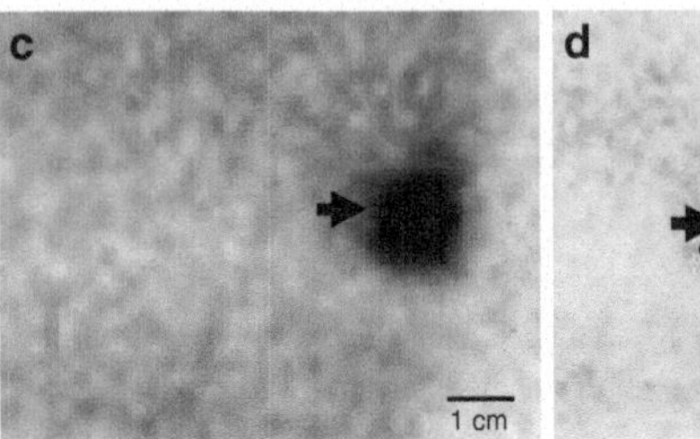
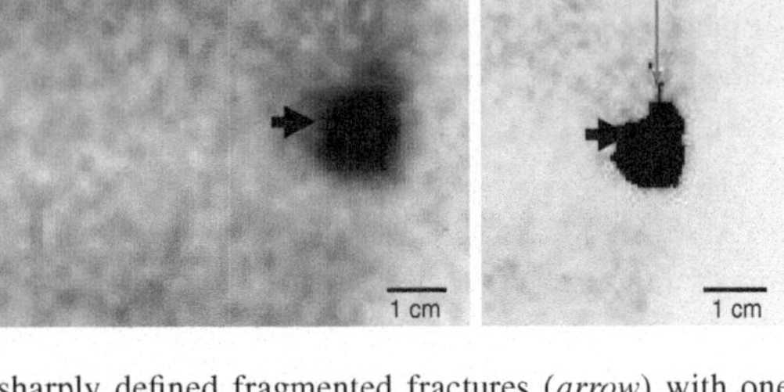

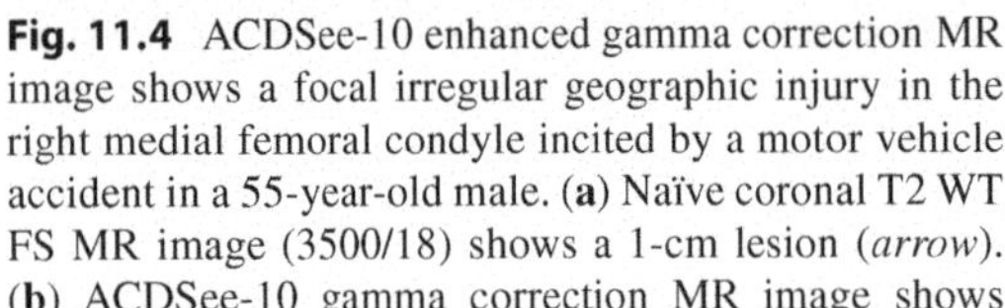

Fig. 11.4 ACDSee-10 enhanced gamma correction MR image shows a focal irregular geographic injury in the right medial femoral condyle incited by a motor vehicle accident in a 55-year-old male. (**a**) Naïve coronal T2 WT FS MR image (3500/18) shows a 1-cm lesion (*arrow*). (**b**) ACDSee-10 gamma correction MR image shows sharply defined fragmented fractures (*arrow*) with one 200 μm microcallus. (**c**) Naïve pinhole scan demonstrates blurry round tracer uptake (*arrow*). (**d**) ACDSee-10 gamma correction view shows sharply defined geographic fracture (*large arrow*) with dash-shaped calluses (*arrow*)

correction pinhole scan findings (Bahk et al. 2017) and H&E stain (Fig. 11.1d, h). Results were that gamma correction MRI showed *15* single-pixelled 200-μm microcalluses and gamma correction pinhole bone scan showed only *five* 200-μm microcalluses. It was confirmed that MRI demonstrability was *three* times higher. Six cases were male and three were female. The age ranged from 15 to 71 years with the average being 38.2. CTMF involved the bones of the shoulder girdle ($n = 2$), hip joint ($n = 1$), knee joint ($n = 3$), ankle ($n = 2$), and foot ($n = 1$). As a model case, a surgically removed femoral head specimen was meticulously analyzed histopathologically to confirm that gamma correction MRI is more efficient and sensitive than ^{99m}Tc-HDP pinhole bone scan for the imaging diagnosis of CTMF although the latter is specific by itself so that it can be used as validation basis. Actually, ACDSee-10 gamma correction MRI very finely imaged CTMF to be precisely measured using a 10× magnifying lens.

11.2 ACDSee-10 Gamma Correction MRI for Demonstration and Pixel Counting of Callused Trabecular Microfracture

Seriated naïve and ACDSee-10 gamma correction ^{99m}Tc-HDP pinhole bone scans were basically performed to validate the diagnosis of trabecular bone changes (Bahk et al. 2017) and the gamma correction was successfully imported to MRI. Naïve coronal T2 FS MRI was taken in each of hereafter presented clinical cases and it was technically processed successively using ACDSee-10 gamma correction to distinctly highlight CTMF (Fig. 11.4). On gamma correction MRI, the bright signal intensity of edema and hemorrhage was suppressed by clicking toolbars in sequence. It is to be remembered that MRI presents callused microfracture in bright signal intensity against black matrix (Fig. 11.4b) and contrary pinhole bone scan presents microfracture in dark ^{99m}Tc-HDP uptake against bright matrix (Fig. 11.4d). The smallest CTMF measured 200 μm in size.

11.3 Sharper Anatomic Display of Trabecular Microfracture by ACDSee-10 Gamma Correction MR Image Compared to Gamma Correction ^{99m}Tc-HDP Pinhole Bone Scan

It is to be remarked that upgraded ACDSee-10 gamma correction MRI can very neatly and sensitively visualize CTMF without penumbra. Actually, ACDSee-10 gamma correction MRI demonstrated as many as *15* single pixel microfractures in nine cases, but ACDSee-10 pinhole bone scan showed only *five*. Theoretically, such an obvious sensitivity difference was presumed to reflect that the image resolution of 2D MRI is threefold higher than that of 3D pinhole bone scan and also to reflect that overall systemic image resolution of MRI is superior compared to that of gamma correction ^{99m}Tc-HDP pinhole bone scan. As already mentioned, however, the gamma correction MRI was disadvantageously unable to provide the osteoneogenetic information like pinhole bone scan does.

11.4 Improved Image of Unit-Pixel Trabecular Fracture by ACDSee-10 Gamma Correction MRI Compared to Gamma Correction ^{99m}Tc-HDP Pinhole Bone Scan

In order to test the fidelity of gamma correction demonstration, we meticulously compared the image resolution of CTMF on ACDSee-10 gamma correction MRI and ^{99m}Tc-HDP pinhole bone scan by counting how many single-pixel microfractures are imaged using each method as illustrated in *nine* clinical cases presented below. Presentations were meant to make a seeing-is-believing account for the unexpectedly raised clinical usefulness of ACDSee-10 gamma correction MRI as an in vivo diagnosis and size measurement tool of CTMF. First, the seriated naïve and gamma correction of MR images was performed and then it was followed by gamma correction ^{99m}Tc-HDP pinhole bone scanning for a validation purpose. The gamma correction used for this investigation was upgraded ACDSee-10 version that can neatly image CTMF without penumbra which prevents precise size measurement.

11.4.1 Case Presentations

Case 1

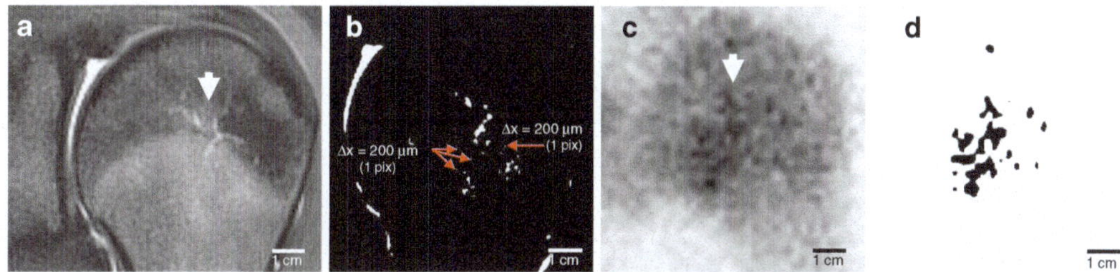

ACDSee-10 gamma correction MR image shows lightning-like branching microfractures in the left humeral head incited by contusion in a 20-year-old male. (**a**) Naïve coronal T2 WT MR image (5,240/70) shows blurry branching fractures (*arrow*). Their localization is central and branching is centrifugal distinguishing it from blood vessels which centripetally distribute. (**b**) Gamma correction MR image distinctly shows four 200-μm pinpointed and few archipelagic callused trabecular microfractures with bright signal intensity. Individual calluses can be accurately imaged and counted and measured in terms of pixel using magnifying optic lens. Δx is number of pixel in the x-axis and Δy in the y-axis. (**c**) Naïve ^{99m}Tc-HDP pinhole bone scan shows nonspecific blurry tracer uptake (*arrow*) (**d**) In contrast, gamma correction pinhole bone scan highlights archipelagic and several neatly defined callused trabecular microfractures with unsuppressed tracer uptake. There is no 200-μm microfracture shown on pinhole bone scan suggesting that MRI would be more sensitive

Case 2

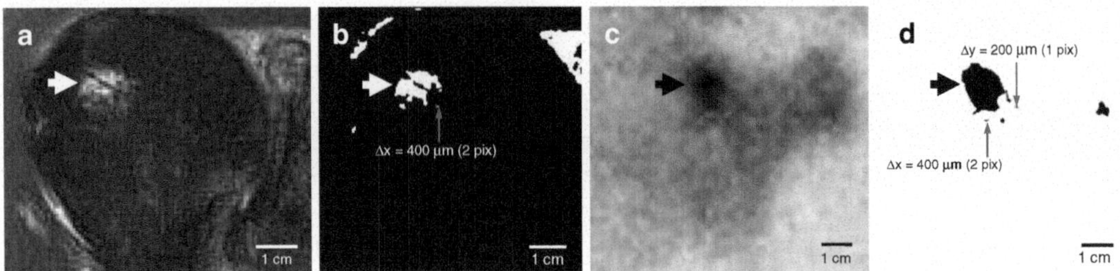

ACDSee-10 gamma correction MRI shows microfractures in the lesser tubercle of the right humerus in a 42-year-old male novice bodybuilder. (**a**) Naïve coronal T2 weighted FS MR image (5,240/70) shows a blurry notched screw-head-like area of bright signal intensity (*arrow*). (**b**) Gamma correction view shows screw-head-like fracture (*white arrow*) with two microfractures the smallest size of which measures 400 μm consisting of 2 pixels (*red arrows*). (**c**) Naïve ^{99m}Tc-HDP pinhole scan shows blurry tracer uptake (*frame*). (**d**) Gamma correction pinhole bone scan shows geographic tracer uptake (*large arrow*) and three distinctly defined unsuppressed microfractures the smallest size of which measured 200 μm in size consisting of single pixel as counted using 10× magnifying lens.

Case 3

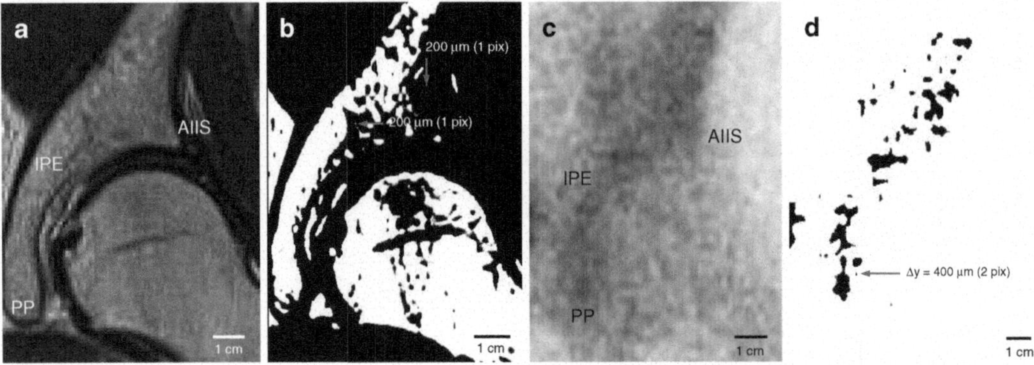

Gamma correction MRI shows a number of pinpointed and speckled microfractures in the left anterior inferior iliac spine (AIIS), ilio-pubic eminence (IPE), and pecten pubis (PP) due to motor vehicle accident in a 30-year-old male. (**a**) Naïve coronal T2 weighted MR image (6000/70) shows nonspecific blurry speckled signal intensity in AIIS, IPE, and PP. (**b**) Gamma correction MR image shows a number of sharply defined speckled and pinpointed fractures with bright signal intensity. There are two 200-μm pinpointed microfractures (*arrows*). (**c**) Naïve ^{99m}Tc-HDP pinhole scan shows nonspecific blurry speckled tracer uptake. (**d**) Gamma correction pinhole scan shows sharply defined microfractures. There is one 400-μm microfracture in the bottom, but no 200-μm microfracture.

Case 4

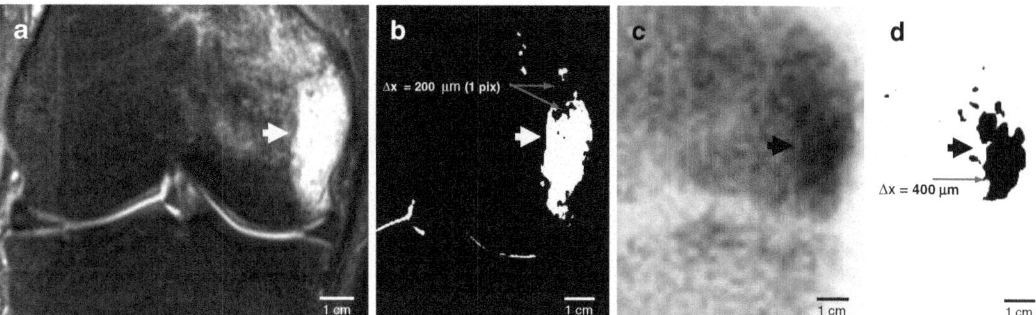

ACDSee-10 gamma correction MRI shows a large ovoid block-like cometary fracture with associated drifting edema in the right medial femoral condyle incited by motor vehicle accident in a 71-year-old male. (**a**) Naïve coronal T2 WT FS MR image (3500/18) shows a 1.3 × 3 cm vertically oriented ovoid fracture with bright signal intensity in cometary fracture with drifting edema (*frame*). (**b**) Gamma correction view shows a large ovoid aggregation of irregular geographic fractures with bright signal intensity (*large arrow*) accompanied by multiple microfractures, three of which were 200 μm in size each involving one pixel (*arrows*). (**c**) Naïve ^{99m}Tc-HDP pinhole scan shows nonspecific blurry tracer uptake (*large arrow*) with drifting edema with lower tracer uptake (*frame*). (**d**) Gamma correction shows the suppression of edema uptake highlighting main fractures (*large arrow*), which is accompanied by microfractures with the smallest one measuring 400 μm (*red arrow*).

Case 5

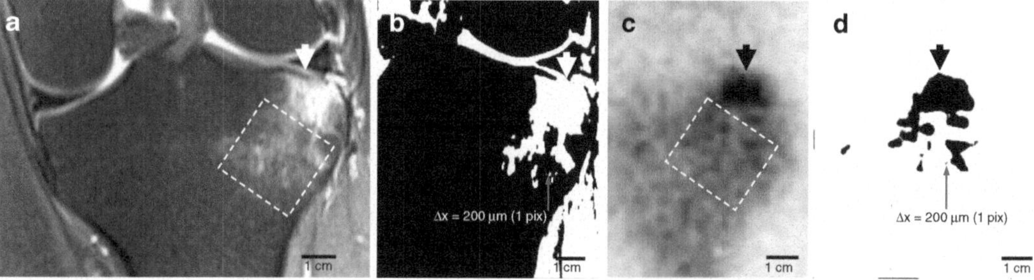

ACDSee-10 gamma correction MRI shows a 1.5-cm irregular cometary fracture with edema in the lateral tibial condyle incited by motor vehicle accident in a 71-year-old male. (**a**) Naïve coronal T2 WT MR image (3,500/18) shows blurry bright signal intensity (*arrow*) with edema in tail (*frame*). (**b**) Gamma correction MRI reveals the suppression of edema highlighting a robot-like fracture with several microfractures with the smallest one measuring 200 μm in size (*arrow*). (**c**) Naïve pinhole scan shows blurry irregular tracer uptake in edema in tail (*frame*). (**d**) Gamma correction pinhole bone scan shows a well defined main fracture (*black arrow*) with a few microfractures. The smallest one involves a single pixel which measures 200 μm in size (*bottom arrow*).

Case 6

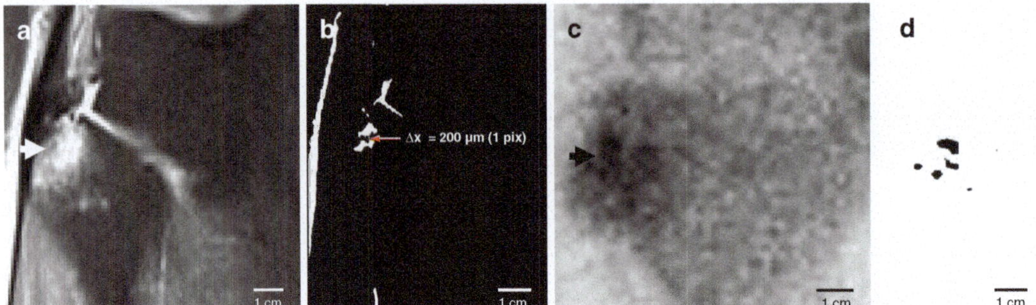

ACDSee-10 gamma correction MRI shows trabecular microfractures in the right fibular head incited by motor vehicle accident in a 64-year-old male. (**a**) Naïve coronal proton density MR image (3,500/18) shows a blurry ovoid fracture (*arrow*) with bright signal intensity. (**b**) Gamma correction MR image shows the suppression of edema and hemorrhage signal highlighting mottled and microfractures with bright signal intensity in microfractures (*arrows*). There is a 200-μm microfracture. (**c**) Naïve ^{99m}Tc-HDP pinhole scan shows nonspecific blurry tracer take (*arrow*) with mottled areas of higher tracer uptake. (**d**) Gamma correction view shows several small mottled fractures but without 200-μm pinpointed one.

Case 7

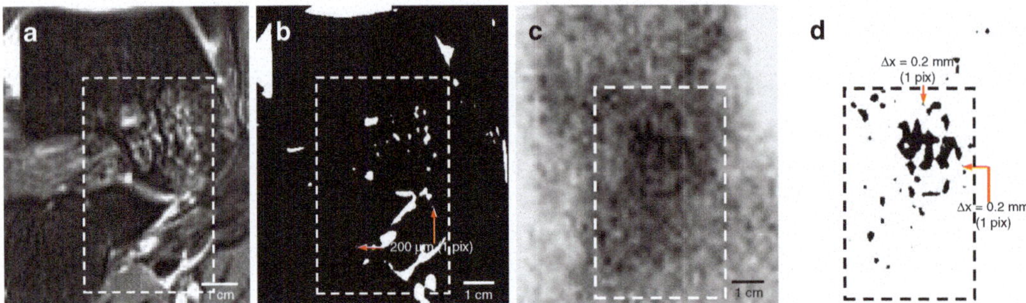

ACDSee-10 gamma correction MRI of inversion sprain of the right ankle shows multiple trabecular microfractures in the talar neck and navicular bone incited by slip down in staircase in a 29-year-old male. (**a**) Naïve coronal proton density FS (2,800/31) MR image shows nonspecific aggregation of blurry pinpointed and speckled bright signal intensity areas in the talar neck and the navicular bone (*frame*). The ankle joint shows synovial effusion with bright signal intensity. (**b**) Gamma correction MR image shows two sharply defined 200-μm microfractures (*frame*). (**c**) Naïve ^{99m}Tc-HDP pinhole bone scan shows nonspecific blurry tracer uptake (*frame*). (**d**) Gamma correction pinhole scan shows the suppression of edema and hemorrhage highlighting large geographic and pinpointed, speckled, and mottled microfractures with unwashed high tracer uptake (*frame*). The smallest fracture involves one single pixel which measures 200 μm in size.

Case 8

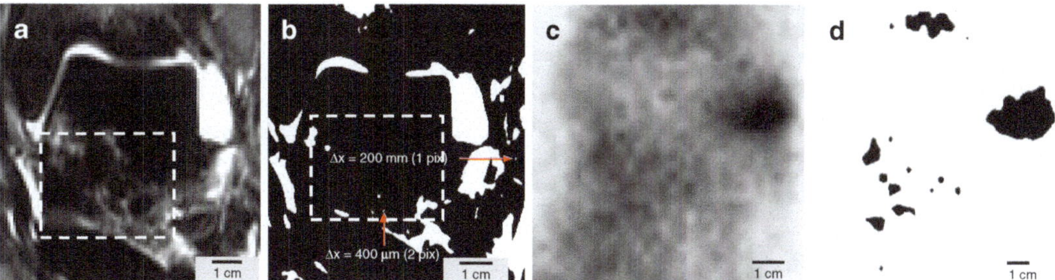

ACDSee-10 gamma correction trabecular microfractures in the neck of the left talus due to strained loop jumping in an 18-year-old female. (**a**) Naïve coronal proton density FS MRI (2800/31) shows nonspecific blurry increased signal intensity in the talar neck (*frame*). The ankle joint shows synovial effusion with bright signal intensity. (**b**) Gamma correction MRI shows speckled unsuppressed bright signal intensity denoting microfractures as observed by a magnifying lens (*frame*). The smallest one was 200 μm in size (*horizontal arrow*). (**c**) Naïve ^{99m}Tc-HDP pinhole scan shows nonspecific blurry tracer uptake (*frame*). (**d**) Gamma correction pinhole scan shows multiple sharply defined speckled fractures but without 200-μm fracture.

Case 9

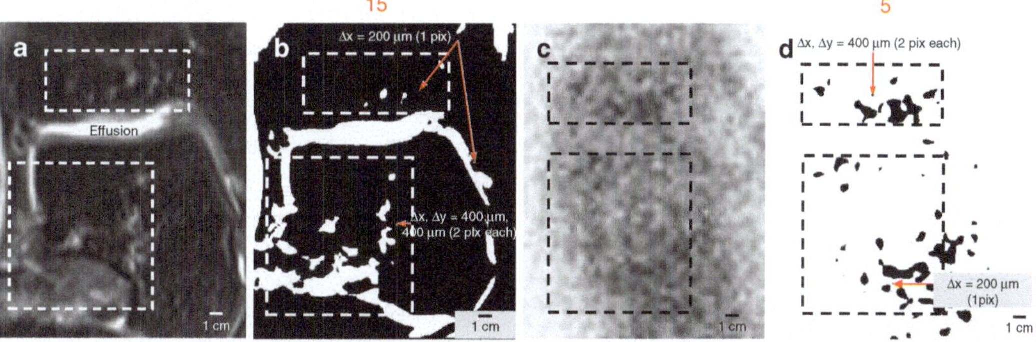

ACDSee-10 gamma correction MRI of the motor-vehicle trodden left hindfoot shows trabecular microfractures in a 15-year-old female. (**a**) Naïve coronal proton density FS MRI (2800/31) shows nonspecific blurry speckled and pinpointed bright signal intensity in the talar neck (*bottom frame*) and the distal tibial epiphysis (*top frame*). There is diffuse synovial effusion in the ankle joint. (**b**) Gamma correction MR image shows two 200-μm microfractures (*top arrow*) and other injuries with highlighted bright signal intensity (frames). (**c**) Naïve ^{99m}Tc-HDP pinhole scan shows nonspecific blurry speckled tracer uptake (*frames*). (**d**) Gamma correction pinhole bone scan demonstrates one 200-μm microfracture and many other neatly defined microfractures (*frames*).

Histologically, trabecular fracture heals by callus formation. The callus is the unorganized meshwork of woven bone developed on the fibrin clot, which will be normally replaced ultimately by hard adult bone. It forms not only to anatomically heal TMF but also to restore marrow spaces for hematopoietic tissues, blood vessels, and fat. Clinically, nontraumatic microfracture can physiologically occur in the presenile population but it may become an important health problem in the aged population (Tassani et al. 1993). CTMF can be imaged and measured using upgraded ACDSee-10 gamma correction ^{99m}Tc-HDP pinhole bone scan (Bahk et al. 2016, 2017) in humans and in vivo in mice using MR image (Haffner-Luntzer et al. 2017). It appears that no in vivo imaging means have been published to specifically demonstrate and clinically diagnose trabecular pathologies including CTMF except for synchrotron radiation micro CT (Okazaki et al.

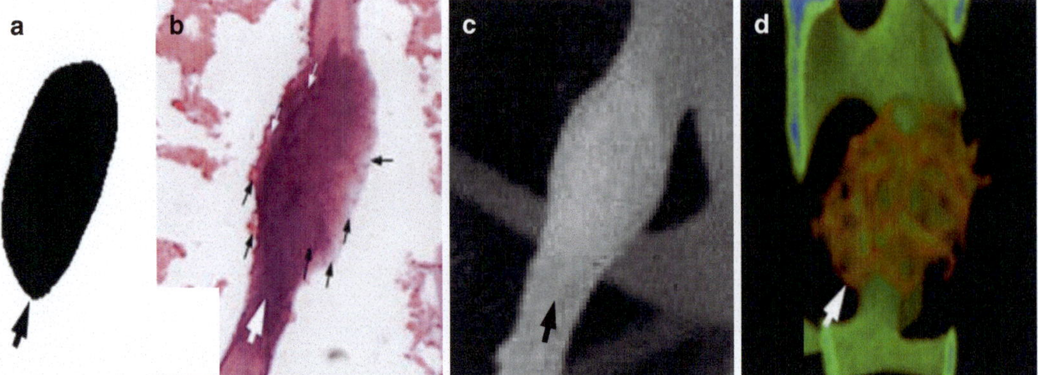

Fig. 11.5 Various image presentations of callused trabecular microfracture. (**a**) In vivo gamma correction ^{99m}Tc-HDP pinhole bone scan. The bone scan image can simultaneously provide bone metabolic information in terms of high or low tracer uptake through unsuppression or suppression using gamma correction. (**b**) H&E stain shows characteristic base stain of osteoneogenesis. (**c**) Cadaveric calloused trabecular microfracture (Vernon-Roberts and Pirie 1973). (**d**) Synchrotron radiation micro CT is useful for metabolic assessment of injured trabeculae, but trabeculae and callused trabecular microfracture appears to be morphologically unnatural and aberrant

2014) that is valuable for the metabolic assessment of injured trabeculae, but thereby attained trabeculae and callused trabeculae appear to be anatomically somewhat aberrant (Fig. 11.5).

As well-known MRI has become to be the most widely used imaging modality for the clinical diagnosis of the diseases of bone and cartilage and joint as well as thereto attached nonosseous supporting tissues such as fibrous joint capsule, ligament, tendon, bursa, and muscle. However, available image would appear to have not yet reached the level to neatly depict and precisely measure the size of CTMF. It is the most basic and smallest bone element injuries to ubiquitously occur in bone trauma, osteoporosis, aseptic osteonecrosis, inflammatory, infective, metabolic, and neoplastic diseases of bone, and even in daily laborious works, sports, and physical stresses. Interestingly, all damaged human body tissues heal by heterogeneous fibroid scar or hypertrophy, but peculiarly enough trabeculae fracture is cured by osteoneogenesis in the form of ossifying callus. As illustrated in case presentations, we recently became to learn that ACDSee-10 can very finely and neatly image CTMF. As such, we carried out this prospective clinical imaging study to import the lately upgraded ACDSee-10 to MRI to cleanly image and quantitate CTMF. Prior to upgrading, we used ACDSee-7 gamma correction for the imaging studies of CTMF (Bahk et al. 2017). Like ACDSee-7, upgraded ACDSee-10 gamma correction can be easily installed in any type of computer to highlight microfracture by suppressing bone marrow edema and hemorrhage, which disturbingly blur MRI signal as it does in ^{99m}Tc-HDP pinhole bone scan (Bahk 2017). Advanced imaging means such as gamma correction ^{99m}Tc-HDP pinhole bone scan and gamma correction MRI have been shown to specifically demonstrate individualized CTMF the size of which can now be measured in terms of pixel involvement using magnifying lens pixel counting method. It is to be emphasized again that the smallest size in terms of number of injured pixel may vary according to the computer model. Ours is 200 μm in size.

The results of the current study in nine consecutive clinical cases confirmed that ACDSee-10 enhanced gamma correction T2 WT MRI of trabecular microfracture can very sharply define and more sensitively demonstrate it than ACDSee-7 which we used in earlier works (Fig. 11.2) (Bahk et al. 2017). The materials we assessed included the bones of the shoulder girdle, hip, knee, ankle, and foot. The diagnosis of CTMF in individual cases made using ACDSee-10 enhanced gamma correction of MRI was meticulously compared to and carefully validated based on the characteristic findings shown by foregoing

ACDSee gamma correction pinhole bone scan and H&E stain (Fig. 11.1) (Bahk et al. 2017). As presented in this model case, we made detailed correlative assessment of the findings of callused TMF revealed by seriated naïve and ACDSee-10 gamma correction pinhole scans, surgical specimen, surface microscopic change, and finally H&E stain. Additionally, the findings of seriated naïve and ACDSee-10 enhanced gamma correction MR images were analyzed in nine consecutive cases. The results indicate that gamma correction MRI can highlight callused TMF through the suppression of blurry edema and hemorrhage, which is verified in each case based on correlative findings of pinhole bone scan and H&E stain. Furthermore, the individual calluses could be precisely measured simply using a 10× magnifying lens as shown in Case Presentations. Technically, there were difficulties in discerning completely injured pixel from incompletely injured pixel with certainty since the brightness of MRI signal and the darkness of bone scan varied from complete to partial or faint. Hence, we arbitrarily decided that pixel was positively injured when MRI signal intensity is "enough bright" on gamma correction MRI and "enough dark" on gamma correction pinhole bone scan.

Interestingly enough, ACDSee-10 enhanced gamma correction MRI showed 15 single-pixelled microfracture, whereas the gamma correction pinhole bone scan showed only five. Such an obvious difference was theoretically presumed to be due to high sensitivity of MRI. This difference is considered to imply that the image resolution of T2 weighted MRI is far superior in diagnostic feasibility of CTMF. The smallest size of unit pixel in our computer screen was 200 μm in the x-axis of coordinate. The diagonal of the computer monitor we used in this study was 24 inches and screen resolution was 1920 × 1080, Samsung LS23C340. Seoul, South Korea.

With rapidly extending longevity and ever encouraged physical activity of aged human being, trabecular microfracture has naturally become not only an important medical but also socioeconomical concern. Fortunately, ACDSee-10 enhanced gamma correction 1.5-tesla MRI can sensitively and specifically diagnose it.

References

Bahk YW. Combined scintigraphic and radiographic diagnosis of bone and joint diseases: including gamma correction interpretation, Chapter 24. 5th ed. Berlin: Springer; 2017. p. 567–648.

Bahk YW, Chung YA, Lee U-Y, et al. Gamma correction ^{99m}hydroxymethylene diphosphonate pinhole bone scan diagnosis and histopathological verification of trabecular contusion in young rats. Nucl Med Commun. 2016;37:988–91.

Bahk YW, Hwang SH, Lee UY, et al. Morphobiochemical diagnosis of acute trabecular microfractures using gamma correction Tc-99m HDP pinhole bone scan with histopathological verification. Medicine. 2017;96(45):e8419.

Dorland's Medical Dictionary. Definition of callus. 32nd ed. Philadelphia, PA: Elsevier Saunders; 2012. p. 273.

Fayad LM, Jacobs MA, Wang X, et al. Musculoskeletal tumors: how to use anatomic, functional, and metabolic MR techniques. Radiology. 2012;265:340–65.

Fazzarali NL. Trabecular microfracture. Calcif Tissue Int. 1993;53(Suppl 1):S143–6.

Frost HM. The spinal osteoporosis: mechanisms of pathogenesis and pathophysiology. Clin Endocrinol Metab. 1973;2:257–75.

Haffner-Luntzer M, Mueller-Graf F, Matthys R, et al. In vivo evaluation of fracture callus development during bone healing in mice using an MRI-compatible osteosynthesis device for mouse femur. J of visualized experiments (jove). 2017; https://doi.org/10.3791/56679.

Jung JY, Cheon GJ, Lee YS, et al. Pixelized measurement of ^{99m}Tc-HDP micro particle formed in gamma correction phantom pinhole scan: a reference study. Nucl Med Mol Imaging. 2016;50:207–12.

Mandalia V, Henson JH. Traumatic bone bruising—a review article. Eur J Radiol. 2008;67:54–61.

McFarland PH, Frost HL. A possible cause for aseptic necrosis of the femoral head. Henry Ford Med Bull. 1961;9:115–22.

Okazaki N, Chiba K, Taguchi K, et al. Trabecular microfractures in the femoral head with osteoporosis: Analysis of microcallus formations by synchrotron radiation micro CT. Bone. 2014;64:82–7.

Partovi S, Tengg-Kobligk H, Bhojwani N, et al. Advanced noncontrast MR imaging in musculoskeletal radiology. Radiol Clin N Am. 2015;53:549–67.

Tassani S, Matsopoulos GK. The micro-structure of bone trabecular fracture: an inter-site study. Bone. 2013;60:78–86.

Vernon-Roberts B, Pirie CJ. Healing trabecular microfractures in the bodies of lumbar vertebrae. Ann Rheum Dis. 1973;32:406–12.

12 ACDSee-10 Gamma Correction Conventional Radiography for Demonstration and Size Measurement of Callused Trabecular Microfracture

Presumably due to rapid, astonishing development of sophisticated modern imaging means such as MRI and MDCT the golden valued conventional radiography seemed to have become unimportantly treated and left behind in this imaging surge. Recently, however, the hitherto undervalued conventional radiographic imaging of bone trabeculae suddenly began to be afresh reappraised in the form of gamma correction radiography. The diagnostic usefulness of naïve conventional radiograph appears to be well comparable to CT and MRI. Basically, we were able to visually confirm the fineness of the image quality of normal trabeculae, for example, in the calcaneus. Morphologically, normal trabeculae were analyzed by simple comparison as they were visualized on conventional radiographs, MDCT, and 1.5 T MRI taken in middle-aged subjects. The lateral image of normal calcaneus showed very fine thready trabeculae in all three imaging modalities (Fig. 12.1). Radiograph showed fine radiopaque linear trabeculae and MDCT showed less fine bright radiopaque trabeculae, while 1.5-T T-2 WT FS MRI showed similar fine trabeculae in dark intensity. The fineness of trabeculae is practically the same in radiograph and MR although the image presentation is bright in radiograph and dark in MRI. It is to be mentioned that the difference in image quality is closely related to the version of imaging machines used. Furthermore, lately introduced upgraded ACDSee-10 gamma correction ^{99m}Tc-HDP pinhole bone scan can very neatly image the injured trabeculae with unsuppressed

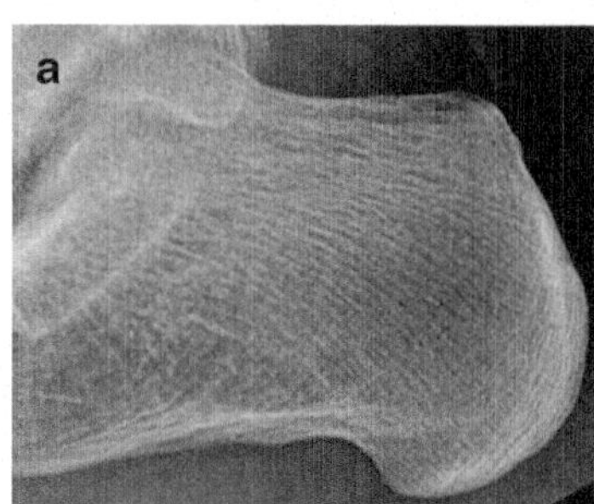

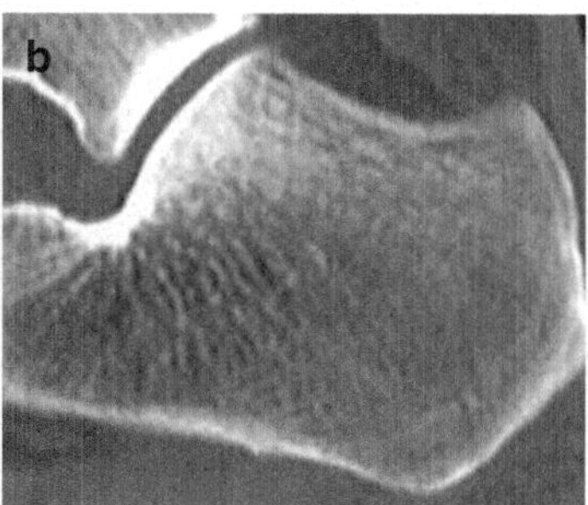

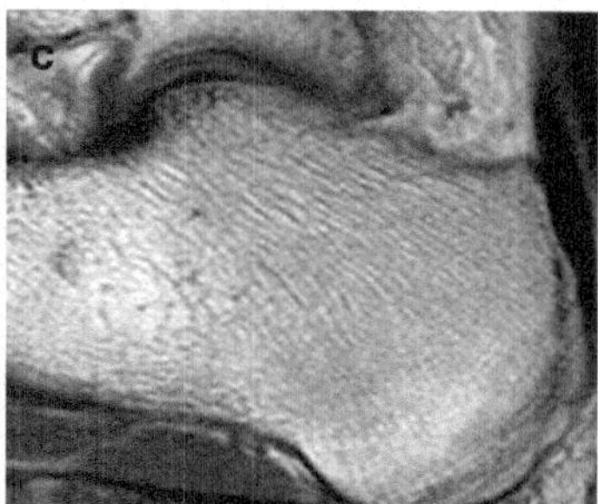

Fig. 12.1 Relative difference of image resolution of normal calcaneal trabeculae shown on the conventional radiograph, MDCT, and 1.5 T MRI in middle-aged subjects. (**a**) The lateral radiograph of normal calcaneus shows fine linear radiopaque (bright) trabeculae. (**b**) MDCT shows less fine trabeculae. (**c**) 1.5-T T-2 WT FS MRI shows fine dark trabeculae. The resolution in terms of sharpness of trabeculae appears to be best in radiograph and MRI

Y.-W. Bahk, *Imaging of Trabecular Microfracture and Bone Marrow Edema and Hemorrhage*,
https://doi.org/10.1007/978-981-15-4466-8_12

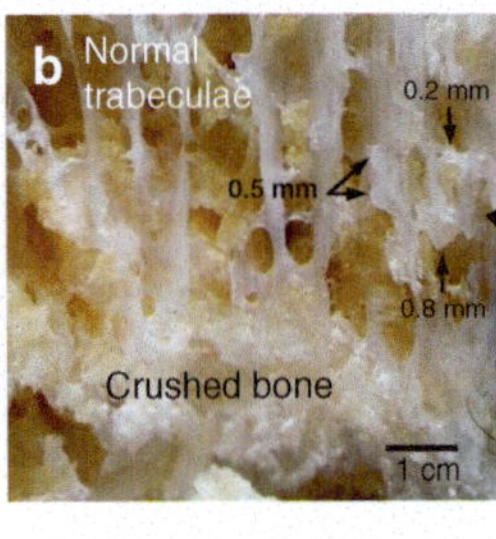

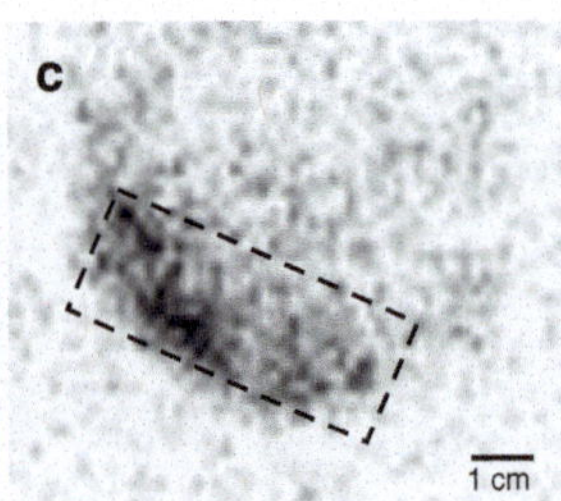

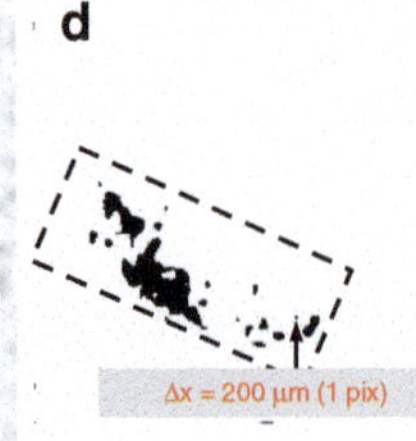

Fig. 12.2 ACDSee-10 gamma correction ^{99m}Tc-HDP pinhole bone scan demonstration and quantitation of the microcalluses formed in trabecular microfractures. (**a**) Surgical specimen shows microcalluses in the femoral neck surface (*frame*). (**b**) Surgical surface microscopy confirms the presence of callused trabecular microfractures and crushed bone as well as normal trabeculae. (**c**) Naïve pinhole bone scan shows nonspecific blurry ^{99m}Tc-HDP uptake (*frame*). (**d**) Gamma correction pinhole bone scan highlights callused trabecular microfractures, the smallest one of which measures 200 μm in size which consists of single pixel

high tracer uptake (Fig. 12.2) (Bahk et al. 2017). Such a distinct demonstration of CTMF naturally drew our attention. The clean imaging of 200-μm sized trabecular microfracture is an important clinical and academic development. Hence, it is fully justified to make a systematic attempt at importing ACDSee-10 gamma correction to the conventional radiograph of CTMF.

This chapter describes the gamma correction method as it is imported to conventional radiography and presents and discusses the results attained from the meticulous analysis of microcalluses observed in consecutive *seven* adult patients including one case each of the shoulder girdle, elbow, wrist, and knee and 3 cases of the hip. Male was three and female was four and ages ranged from 17 to 57 years with the average being 37. Plain bone radiograph of each case was taken using Aristos radiographic system, Siemens, Erlangen, Germany. Image characteristics are 3000 × 3000 = 9,000,000 pixels resolution, pixel size is 143 μm, and depth is 14 bit. The usefulness of gamma correction conventional radiograph was fully validated using gamma correction ^{99m}Tc-HDP bone scanning and histological studies (Fig. 12.3). This is a model case of ACDSee-10 gamma correction conventional radiograph showing the microfractures in the right femoral neck fracture incited by falling down in shower room in a 72-year-old female: Naïve radiograph shows femoral neck fracture with mottled increased densities (*frame*). Gamma correction radiograph shows multiple twin-pixelled 0.4-mm pinpointed calluses (*frame*). Naïve ^{99m}Tc-HDP pinhole scan shows nonspecific blurry tracer uptake (*frame*). ACDSee-7 gamma correction ^{99m}Tc-HDP pinhole scan shows archipelagic fractures with a number of pinpointed calluses. Microfracture is measured using the pixelization method (Jung et al. 2016), fresh surgically removed humeral head showed the broken surface with roughened microfractures that were anatomically confirmed and histologically proven by H&E stain.

Callused trabecular microfractures (Courtesy of Prof. Jin Kim, Department of Anatomy, the Catholic University Medical School, Seoul). Seven Case Presentations will follow (Vide infra).

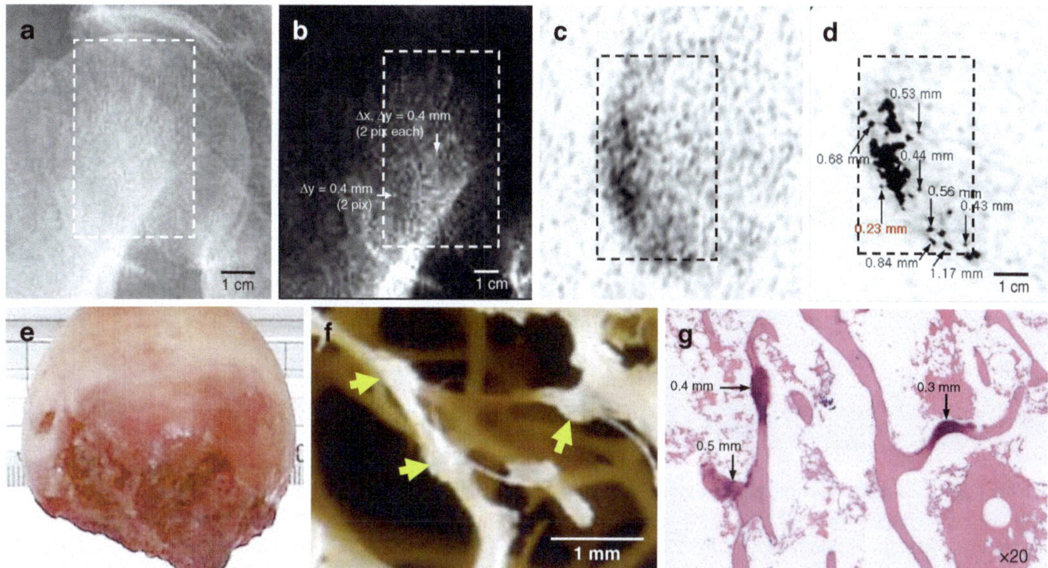

Fig. 12.3 ACDSee—7 gamma correction radiograph shows microfractures in the right humeral head incited by falling down in a shower room in a 72-year-old female. (**a**) Naïve radiograph shows a faintly visible femoral neck fracture with mottled increased trabecular in the femoral head (*frame*). (**b**) Gamma correction radiograph shows multiple twin-pixel 0.4-mm pinpointed fractures (*frame*). (**c**) Naïve pinhole scan shows nonspecific blurry tracer uptake in fractures (*frame*). (**d**) Gamma correction pinhole scan shows archipelagic fractures with multiple microfractures, the size of which is measured using pixelization method (Jung et al. 2016). (**e**) Fresh surgically removed humeral head shows fracture surface with rough microfractures. (**f**) Callused trabecular microfractures (Courtesy of Anatomy Professor Dr. Jin Kim, Catholic University Medical School, Seoul). (**g**) H&E stain shows typical base stained callused trabecular microfractures

12.1 Case Presentations

Case 1

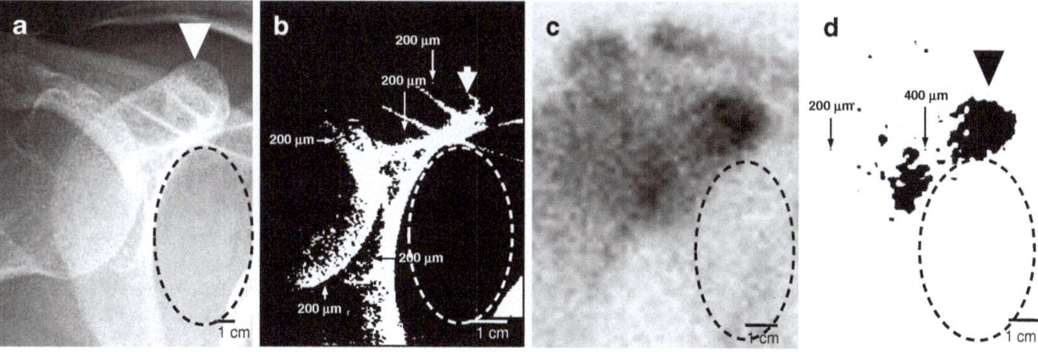

ACDSee-10 gamma correction conventional radiograph of the coracoid process and head of the right humerus shows callused trabecular microfractures incited by a motor vehicle accident in a 33-year-old female. (**a**) Naive radiograph is negative (*arrow*). No trabeculae exist in the infraspinous portion of the scapula because it is a thin compact bone (*circle*). (**b**) Gamma correction radiograph (gamma = −75/0/0) shows an aggregation of 200-µm callused pinpoint trabecular microfractures in the contused coracoid process (*arrows*). (**c**) Naïve ^{99m}Tc-HDP pinhole scan demonstrates increased tracer uptake in the coracoid process and humeral head (*arrow*). (**d**) Gamma correction pinhole scan (gamma = 1/0/0) validates two large geographic and multiple 200- and 400-µm pinpoint trabecular fractures (*arrows*).

Case 2

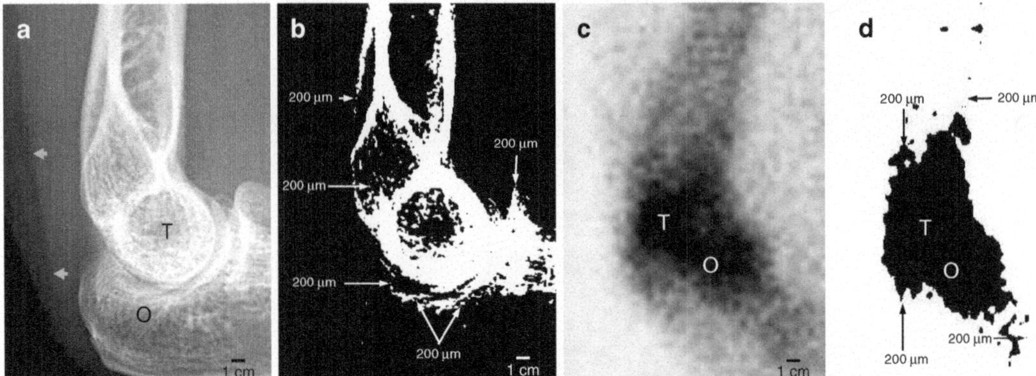

ACDSee-10 gamma correction conventional radiograph demonstrates a large callused geographic and multiple microfractures in the right elbow involving the olecranon (O) and trochlea (T) in a 42-year-old female. This elbow was trapped and injured between the closing door. (**a**) Naïve lateral radiograph shows suspicious trabecular thickening in the trochlea and diffuse swelling of the triceps muscle, tendon, and subcutaneous soft tissue (*arrows*). (**b**) Gamma correction radiograph shows numerous callused trabecular microfractures in the trochlea and olecranon (*arrows;* gamma = –60/0/0). (**c**) Naïve lateral ^{99m}Tc-HDP pinhole scan shows blurry aggregation of irregular mottled hot areas in the trochlea and olecranon. (**d**) Gamma correction (gamma = 1/0/0) pinhole scan shows a large unsuppressed geographic tracer uptake and multiple CTMF with the smallest one measuring 200 µm in size.

Case 3

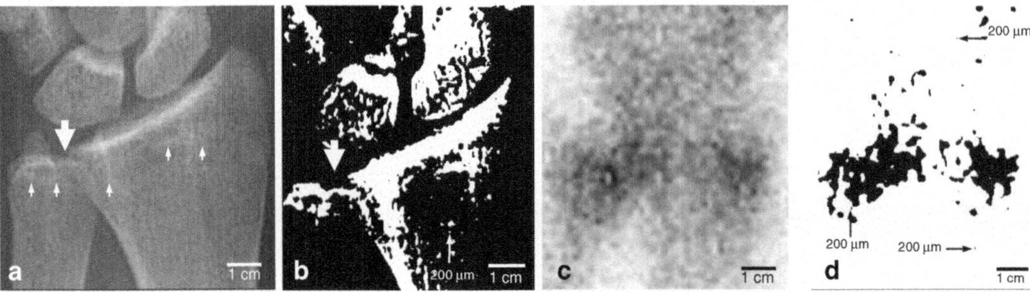

ACDSee-10 gamma correction conventional radiographic demonstration of speckled and pinpointed microfractures of the left distal radial and ulnar epiphyses with mild separation of radioulnar syndesmosis due to motor vehicle wheel treading in a 17-year-old male motor cyclist. (**a**) Naïve radiograph shows separation of the distal radioulnar syndesmosis (*large arrow*) with small faint fluffy lesions (*small arrows*). (**b**) Gamma correction (gamma = -10/0/0) radiograph shows sharply defined speckled and pinpoint microfraccures (*small arrows*) with separation of the distal radioulnar syndemosis (*arrow*). (**c**) Naïve pinhole scan shows nonspecific blurred speckled tracer uptake in the distal ends of the radius and ulna and radioulnar sysndesmosis (*arrows*). (**d**) Gamma correction (gamma = 1/0/0) view shows suppression of edema and hemorrhage highlighting speckled and pinpoint microfractures the smallest one of which measures 200 µm (*arrows*).

Case 4

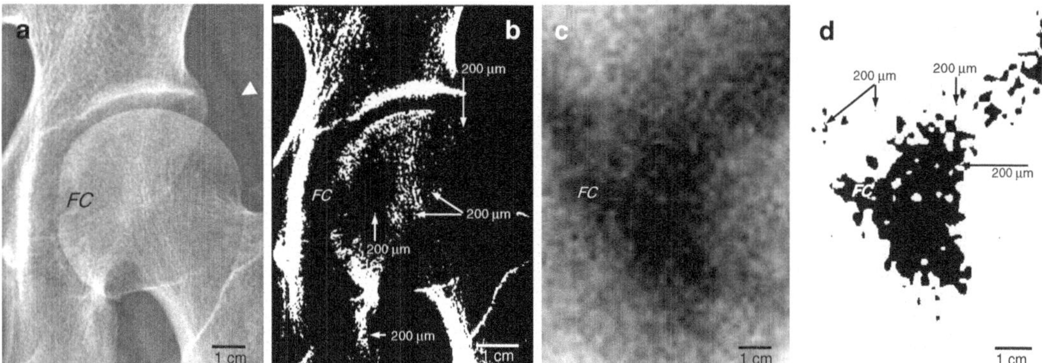

ACDSee-10 gamma correction radiograph shows subchondral trabecular microfractures in the left hip joint bones due to early osteoarthritis in a 46-year-old female. (**a**) Naïve AP radiograph shows osteoporosis of hip joint bones including the acetabulum and fovea capitis (*FC*) with synovitis. (**b**) Gamma correction (gamma = −12/0/0) view demonstrates numerous pinpoint trabecular microfractures mainly in the femoral head (*frame*) due to degenerative osteochondropathy. (**c**) Naïve anterior ^{99m}Tc-HDP pinhole scan shows nonspecific blurry high ^{99m}Tc-HDP uptake (*frame*). (**d**) ACDSee-10 gamma correction view (gamma = −100/−39/−31) highlights unsuppressed reticular and pinpoint high tracer uptake in the foveola capitis (*FC*) and acetabular fossa (*frame*). The smallest fracture measures 200 μm in size.

Case 5

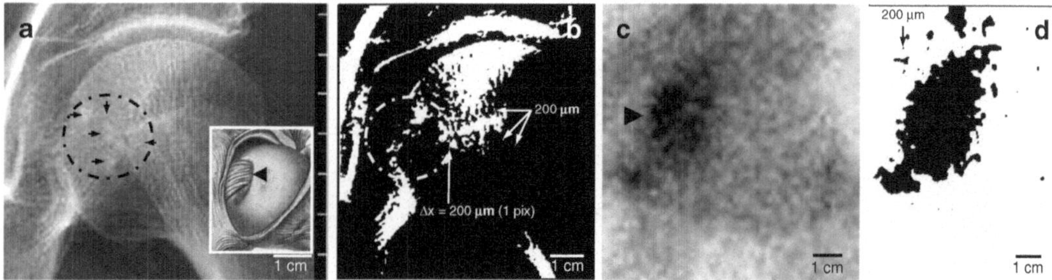

ACDSee-10 gamma correction radiograph of painful chronic calcified microfractures due to trauma are shown in the left femoral head including the fovea capitis in a 32-year-old female. (**a**) Naïve radiograph shows multiple speckled calcifications in the fovea capitis (*circled*). Inset is anatomy of the fovea and ligament (*arrow*) (Clement's Anatomy. Urban & Schwarzenberg, München, 1981). (**b**) Gamma correction (gamma = −74/0/0) view shows microfractures (*arrows*). (**c**) Naïve anterior ^{99m}Tc-HDP pinhole scan shows nonspecific blurry tracer uptake (*arrow*) in the left femoral head. (**d**) Gamma correction (gamma = −7/0/0) view shows fractures with unsuppressed tracer (*frame*). The smallest microfracture measures 200 μm in size.

Case 6

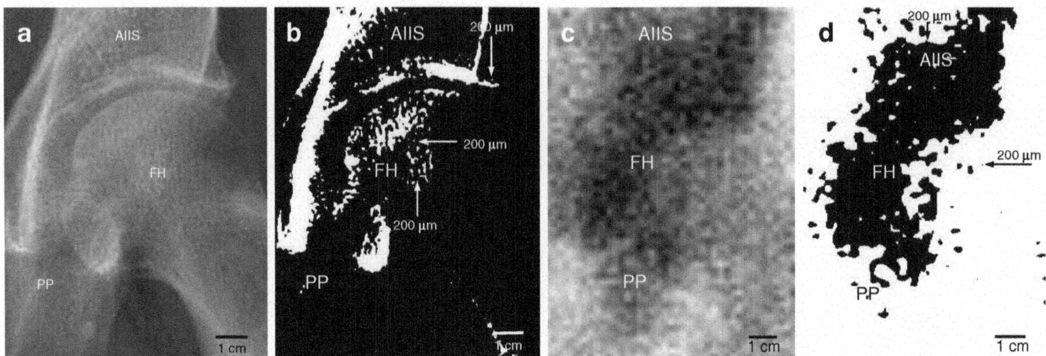

ACDSee-10 gamma correction radiographic demonstration of callused microfractures in the left hip joint bones including the anterior iliac spine (AIIS), femoral head (FH), and pecten pubis (PP) due to motor vehicle accident in a 32-year-old male. (**a**) Naïve anterior radiograph shows blurry trabeculae. (**b**) Gamma correction (gamma = −50/0/0) radiograph shows multiple 200 μm callused pinpoint trabecular fractures (*arrows*) in AIIS, FH, and PP. (**c**) Naïve anterior ^{99m}Tc-HDP pinhole scan shows nonspecific blurry ^{99m}Tc-HDP uptake in AIIS, FH, and PP. (**d**) Gamma correction (gamma = 7/0/0) suppresses blurry edema and hemorrhage uptake highlighting pinpointed and speckled microfractures in AIIS, FH, and PP. The smallest fractures measure 200 μm in size.

Case 7

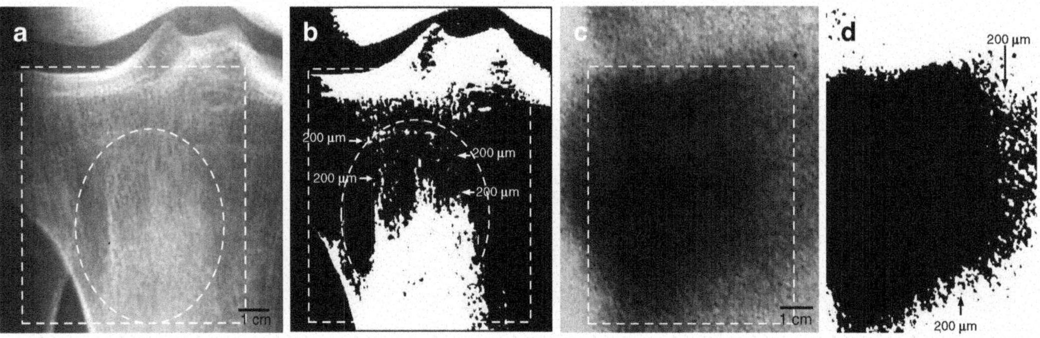

ACDSee-10 gamma correction radiographic demonstration of trabecular microcalluses formed in the right tibial tuberosity incited by motor vehicle contusion in a 57-year-old male. (**a**) Naïve radiograph shows thinning (*frame*) and condensation (*circle*) of trabeculae. (**b**) Gamma correction (gamma = −65/0/0) radiograph shows a large compact aggregation of trabecular fractures along with scattered pinpoint microfractures (*circle*). (**c**) Naïve anterior ^{99m}Tc-HDP pinhole bone scan shows a large blurry area of intense tracer uptake obscuring detail (*frame*). (**d**) Gamma correction (gamma = −35/0/0) suppresses edema and hemorrhage uptake highlighting large unsuppressed tracer uptake with intermixed callused trabecular microfractures. The smallest microfracture measures 200 μm in size.

In conclusion, this chapter has described the rationales, method, and results of gamma correction as it is applied to most basic and popular conventional radiography and presented and discussed the results attained from the meticulous analysis of microcalluses observed in consecutive seven adult patients. Bones studied included one case each of the shoulder girdle, elbow, wrist, and knee and three cases of the hip. Male was three and female was four and ages ranged from 17 to 57 years (average = 37). Conventional radiograph of each case was taken using Aristos radiographic system, Siemens, Erlangen, Germany. Image characteristics were 3000 × 3000 = 9,000,000 pixels resolution, pixel size was 143 μm, and depth was 14 bit. The diagnosis and usefulness of gamma correction radiograph were fully validated using gamma correction ^{99m}Tc-HDP bone scan reinforced by histolopathogical studies.

References

Bahk YW, Hwang S-H, Lee UY, et al. Morophobiochemical diagnosis of acute trabecular microfractures using gamma correction Tc-99m HDP pinhole bone scan with histopathological verification. Medicine. 2017;96:45. (e8419)

Jung J-Y, Cheon GJ, Lee Y-S, et al. Pixelized measurement of ^{99m}Tc-HDP micro particles formed in gamma correction phantom pinhole scan: a reference study. Nucl Med Mol Imaging. 2016;50:207–12.

13 ACDSee-10 Gamma Correction Multidetector Computed Tomographic Demonstration and Quantitation of Callused Trabecular Microfracture

Computed tomography (CT) consists of an X-ray generator, X-ray detector, and computerized imaging and recording systems. The latest model of multidetector computed tomography (MDCT) uses a rotating fan anode of X-ray beams, fixed ring of radiation detectors, and collimator. Human body tissues such as bone and joint and muscle and tendon as well as the brain, lung, and heart and a number of abdominal organs are important objectives of CT examination. Technically, CT computer can convert the X-ray beam attenuation of normal and diseased bone tissues mathematically into a CT number (Hounsfield unit = HU) by comparing it with the X-ray attenuation of H_2O. The attenuation of air is designated to range from −400 to 1000 HU, fat tissue from −60 to −100 HU, body fluid from +20 to +30 HU, muscle from +40 to +80 HU, trabecular bone from +100 to +300 HU, and the attenuation of cortical bone is +1000 HU (Greenspan and Beltran 2015).

Although MDCT, like MRI, lately has become to diagnose malfunctions and anatomic diseases of most organs and tissues in human body including the vital organs such as the thinking brain, constantly beating heart, and ceaselessly respiring lung, in particular, MDCT appears to be relatively attentively used in the skeletal system (Vanhoenacker et al. 2007). However, the further extended application of the ACDSee-10 gamma correction to MDCT also suddenly opened a new avenue to precisely visualize callused trabecular microfracture (CTMF) as gamma-corrected ^{99m}Tc-HDP pinhole bone scan, MRI, and conventional radiography do. The smallest microfracture so demonstrated measured 200 μm in size as presented in earlier chapters. For technical information, the original image resolution of standard pinhole bone scan is 6.2 mm in E-cam gamma camera system of Siemens, Knoxville, Illinois, USA. Following gamma correction, the bone scan image resolution became to be amazingly and wizardly reduced to 200 μm (Fig. 13.1). Thus, it was considered to be worthy of importing ACDSee-10 gamma correction to MDCT to specifically image CTMF as a potent *micrographic imaging tool*. Advantageously, gamma correction is very economical indeed to perform. This chapter presents and discusses the results attained by the analysis of five cases of the acute trabecular microfracture in adult patients including one case each of elbow, lumbar vertebra, femoral neck, and foot and two cases of the knee. Male was 5 and female was 1 and ages ranged from 19 to 92 years with the average being 48.1 years. Each case was examined using ACDSee-10 gamma correction. Technically, ACDSee-10 has been recently upgraded from ACDSee-7 and consequently, we analytically checked the difference of two different versions using ^{99m}Tc-HDP pinhole bone scans. The results proved that ACDSee 7 suffers from blurry penumbra and lower sensitivity and ACDSee 10 version neatly eliminates penumbra and significantly

Y.-W. Bahk, *Imaging of Trabecular Microfracture and Bone Marrow Edema and Hemorrhage*,
https://doi.org/10.1007/978-981-15-4466-8_13

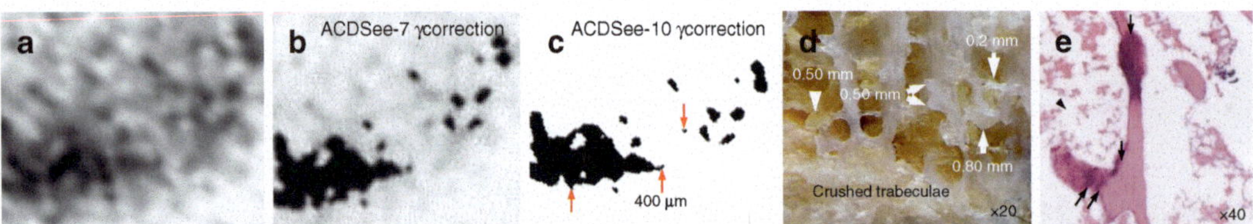

Fig. 13.1 Neater definition and higher sensitivity of ACDSee-10 gamma correction image compared to conventional ACDSee-7 gamma correction with histological validation in surgically removed femoral head for prosthesis in a 72-year-old female patient. (**a**) Naïve ^{99m}Tc-HDP pinhole scan shows nonspecific blurry tracer uptake. (**b**) ACDSee-7 gamma correction pinhole scan shows microcalluses and archipelagic fractures with unsuppressed blurry contour because of penumbra. (**c**) ACDSee-10 gamma correction view shows a sharpened microfracture contour (*red arrows*). Smaller microfractures are shown because of higher image sensitivity. (**d**) Surface microscope of ROI in surgical specimen shows seed-pearly trabecular microfractures and a large crushed trabeculae. (**e**) H&E stain shows callused microfractures with typical base stain

enhances sensitivity. As a matter of fact, the upgraded latter version can very sharply and more sensitively demonstrate 200-μm callused trabecular microfractures. This study was validated using surgical microscopy and H&E stain as shown in Fig. 13.1.

The usefulness of ACDSee-10 gamma correction ^{99m}Tc-HDP pinhole bone scanning, gamma correction MRI, and conventional radiography for the unprecedented micrographic demonstration of callused trabecular microfracture was separately presented and discussed above and now the final turn has come to MDCT. The *MDCT* was first introduced in 1998, and it has become one of the most sophisticated and widely used imaging means for the diagnosis of the skeletal system in the last decade. MDCT makes good use of X-ray and is highly developed imaging technology. Its covering scope is nearly all visceral organs in human body including the incessantly beating heart and ceaselessly respiring lung and all static tissues (Ulzheimer and Flohr 2009). Multislice CT. third ed. Springer-Verlag Berlin-Heidelberg 2009], but not including callused trabecular microfractures the smallest size of which measures 200 μm.

Technically, we were able to image microfractures using seriated naive and ACDSee-10 gamma correction MDCT in six consecutive cases as will be presented below. The usefulness of ACDSee-10 gamma correction MDCT diagnosis was verified in each case using the corroboratory microfracture findings of ACDSee-10 ^{99m}Tc-HDP pinhole bone scan. Results were that the bright CT signal intensity of microfracture was highlighted and precisely measured by directly counting the number of injured pixel by magnifying lens. The injured pixel was characteristically presented as bright CT density against dark background matrix on ACDSee-10 gamma correction CT and conversely dark microscopic ^{99m}Tc-HDP uptake against bright matrix on ACDSee 10 gamma correction pinhole bone scan (Cases 1–6; vide infra). ^{99m}Tc-HDP pinhole bone scan finding was used for the validation of gamma correction MDCT findings of microfracture because unsuppressed high tracer uptake denotes active osteoneogenesis. As mentioned, the smallest size of the unit pixel shown in our computer was 200 μm in the *x*-axis. Generally, ACDSee-10 gamma correction MDCT showed a number of single-pixel trabecular microfractures and the difference was presumed to be due to high sensitivity of CT. The diagonal of computer monitor used in this study was 24 inches and screen resolution was 1920 × 1080, Samsung LS23C340, Seoul, South Korea.

13.1 Case Presentation

Case 1

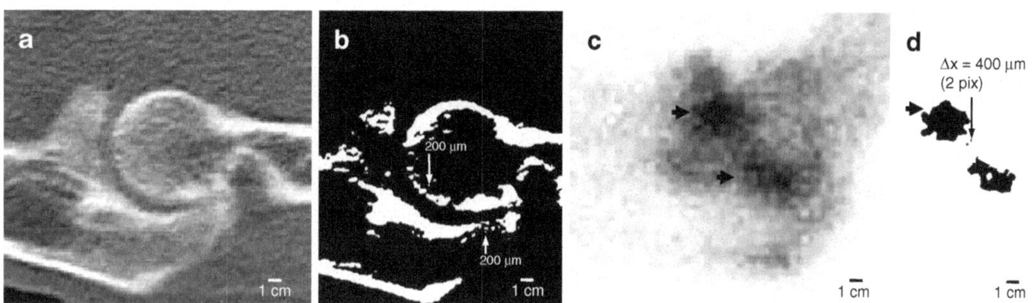

ACDSee-10 gamma correction MDCT of the sprained left elbow in a 49-year-old male demonstrates callused trabecular microfractures. (**a**) Naïve lateral view MDCT shows no bony abnormality. (**b**) Gamma correction MDCT, however, distinctly demonstrates multiple irregular trabecular fractures with high (bright) CT density. The smallest ones measure 200 μm in size. (**c**) Naive ^{99m}Tc-HDP pinhole bone scan shows nonspecific blurry tracer uptake which is nonspecific (*arrows*). (**d**) In contrast, however, gamma correction scan shows drastic change now distinctly revealing archipelagic and few microtrabecular fractures with unsuppressed tracer uptake. It measures 400 μm. ^{99m}Tc-HDP pinhole bone scan was used for validation of the gamma correction MDCT findings.

Case 2

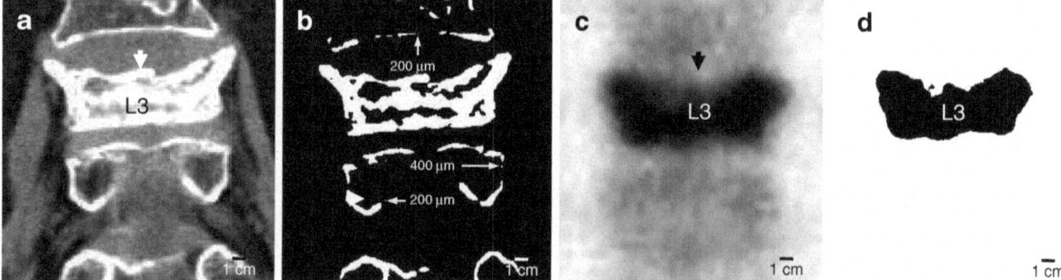

ACDSee-10 gamma correction MDCT for the diagnosis of compression fracture of L3 vertebral body in a 30-year-old male. (**a**) MDCT of L3 vertebra demonstrates roughened compression fracture. (**b**) Gamma correction CT demonstrates compression fracture with two 200- and one 400-μm microcalluses in the L2 lower endplate and L4 vertebra. (**c**) Naïve anterior ^{99m}Tc-HDP pinhole scan shows nonspecific intense tracer uptake with the compression of the upper endplate (*arrow*). (**d**) Gamma correction pinhole bone scan shows a sharply defined L3 upper endplate compression fracture. There is a multipixel small fracture. Observe very sharp delineation of gamma correction MDCT of L3 vertebral compression fracture.

Case 3

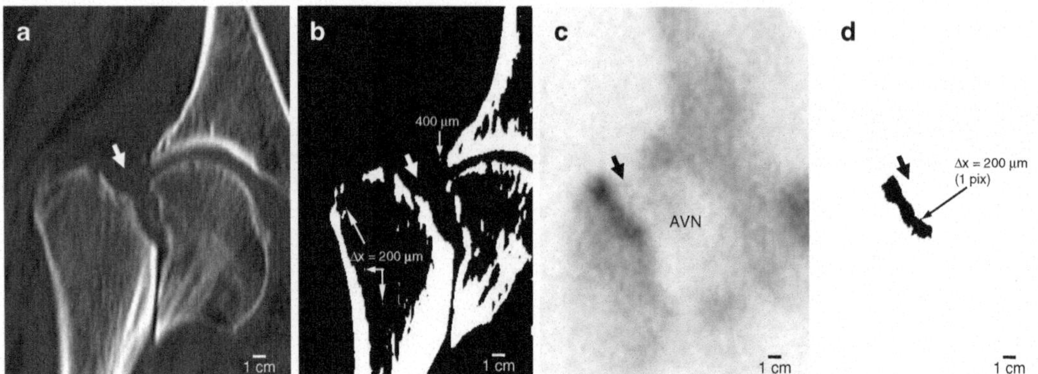

Vertical tearing fracture occurred in the right femoral neck in a 92-year-old male. (**a**) Naïve anteroposterior MDCT of the right hip shows gaping femoral neck fracture (*arrow*). (**b**) ACDSee-10 gamma correction CT shows the main fracture with several 200-μm callused trabecular microfractures (*arrows*). (**c**) Naïve ^{99m}Tc-HDP pinhole scan shows avascular bone necrosis of the femoral head with focal bar-like tracer uptake in the greater tuberosity (*arrow*). (**d**) ACDSee-10 gamma correction bone scan shows a fracture with a 200-μm fracture (*arrow*).

Case 4

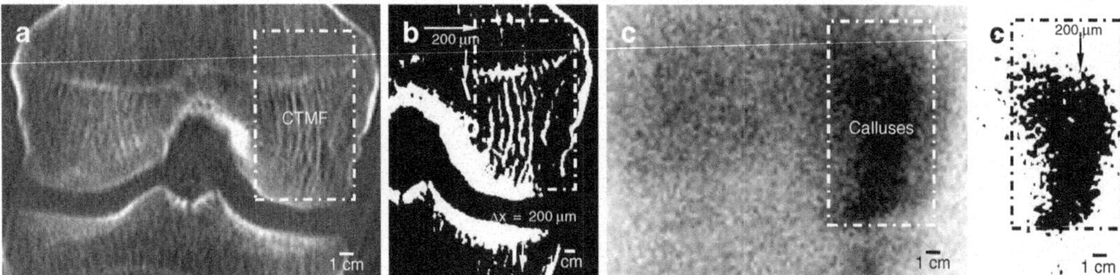

Contusion to the left lateral femoral condyle by motor vehicle in a 71-year-old female (*arrow*). (**a**) Naïve anterior MDCT shows coarsened trabeculae in the lateral femoral condyle (*frame*). (**b**) ACDSee-10 gamma correction MDCT demonstrates coarsened trabeculae with a few 200-μm callused trabecular microcalluses (*frame*). (**c**) Naïve anterior ^{99m}Tc-HDP pinhole scan shows nonspecific blurry tracer uptake in the lateral femoral condyle (*frame*). (**d**) ACDSee-10 gamma correction pinhole scan shows suppression of edema highlighting injured trabeculae including 200-μm microcallus.

Case 5

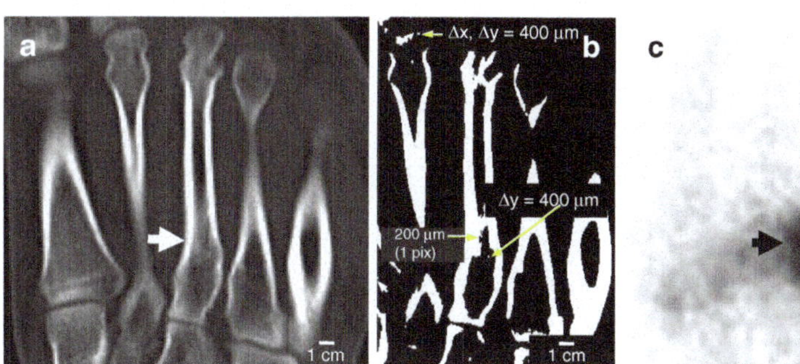

MDCT of the right foot metatarsal bones shows a small vertically oriented radiolucent linear fracture in the proximal portion of the third toe by trauma in a 19-year-old male. (**a**) Naïve MDCT shows a small linear fracture (*arrow*). (**b**) ACDSee-10 gamma correction MDCT demonstrates multiple neatly defined 200-µm microfractures (*arrows*). (**c**) Naïve dorsal 99mTc-HDP pinhole bone scan shows nonspecific blurry tracer uptake (*arrow*). (**d**) However, ACDSee-10 gamma correction pinhole scan neatly demonstrates a peanut-shaped callus with a 400-µm microfracture in the top (*red arrow*).

It is concluded that ACDSee-10 gamma correction MDCT can efficiently demonstrate the callused trabecular microfracture which measures as small as 200 µm in size exactly like gamma correction ^{99m}Tc-HDP pinhole bone scan, MRI, and conventional radiograph. Pinhole bone scan was used for the validation of trabecular microfractures as in MRI.

References

Greenspan A, Beltran J. Computed tomography in introduction to orthopedic imaging. In: Greenspan A, Beltran J, editors. Orthpedic imaging. 6th ed. Philadelphia: Wolters; 2015.

Ulzheimer S, Flohr T. Multislice CT: current technology and future developments. In: Reiser MF, Becker CR, Nikolaou K, Glazer G, editors. Multislice CT. 3rd ed. Berlin Heidelberg: Springer; 2009. p. 3–24.

Vanhoenacker FM, Maas D, Gieln JL. Imaging of orthopedic sports injuries. In: Baert AL, Brady LW, Heilmann HP, editors. Medical radiology. Berlin Heidelberg pp: Springer-Verlag; 2007. p. 95–6.

14 Morphobiochemical Diagnosis of Callused Trabecular Microfracture Using Gamma Correction ^{99m}Tc-HDP Pinhole Bone Scan with Histological Validation

Callused trabecular microfracture (CTMF) ubiquitously occurs in osteoporosis (Vernon-Roberts and Pirie 1973), bone contusion [Mandalia and Henson], aseptic bone necrosis (McFarland and Frost 1961), inflammatory, metabolic, and neoplastic bone diseases (Bahk 2013) and even normal physiological activities (Fazzalari 1993; Frost 1973). Its clinical effect may be negligible when localized. However, if systemic it may become a condition to clinically derange the equilibrium state of the whole skeletal system manifesting not only as a major debilitating disease but also as a serious welfare and socioeconomic problem in aged populations (Tassani and Matsopoulos 2013. Trabecular microfracture heals by microcallus formation, an aggregation of woven bone, presenting as "nodular, fusiform, angulated, or arched bridge lesions" (Fazzalari 1993). We performed this prospective gamma correction ^{99m}Tc-HDP pinhole bone scan study to specifically demonstrate and diagnose trabecular microfractures. The result showed that high tracer uptake in CTMF is unsuppressed by gamma correction, whereas low and moderate tracer uptake in edema and hemorrhage is cleanly suppressed (Bahk 2013). For this gamma correction ^{99m}Tc-HDP pinhole bone scan study, we used devitalized femoral head surgically removed for arthroplasty in six patients. All patients signed informed consent and it was approved by the Institutional Review Board. The preoperative diagnosis of femoral neck fracture was made in all patients by radiography and pinhole bone scan (Fig. 14.1 top panel). The pinhole scans were scrutinized and findings were histopathologically validated. The presence of trabecular microfractures was confirmed in Cases 1–3 and strongly suggested in 4–6 by base stain (Fig. 14.1 bottom panel).

Historically, trabecular microfracture began to draw attention of researchers in the early 1960s as they were found in the necrotized femoral head in patients with hypercortisonism (McFarland and Frost 1961). In the beginning, it was studied using conventional radiography which was then replaced by MR. The value of MRI for the diagnosis of TMF was first reported by Yao and Lee (1988). They observed high signal intensity in the T2-weighted image and speckled or linear low signal intensity in the T1-weighted image in contused knee bones. These results were confirmed and furthered in a larger number of patients by Mink and Deutch (1989). On the other hand, Rangger et al. (1998) performed a histological investigation of trabecular microfractures using cryosection and Ryu et al. (2000) studied the MRI findings of a bone contusion in swine. Recently, micro-computed tomography (micro CT) (Ito 2011; Okazaki et al. 2014; Klinstrom, et al. 2014) and micro magnetic resonance imaging (micro MRI) (Song and Wehrli 1999; Rajapakse et al. 2012) were developed for the 3D imaging of trabecular microfracture. In addition, our group found that ^{99m}Tc-HDP

Y.-W. Bahk, *Imaging of Trabecular Microfracture and Bone Marrow Edema and Hemorrhage*,
https://doi.org/10.1007/978-981-15-4466-8_14

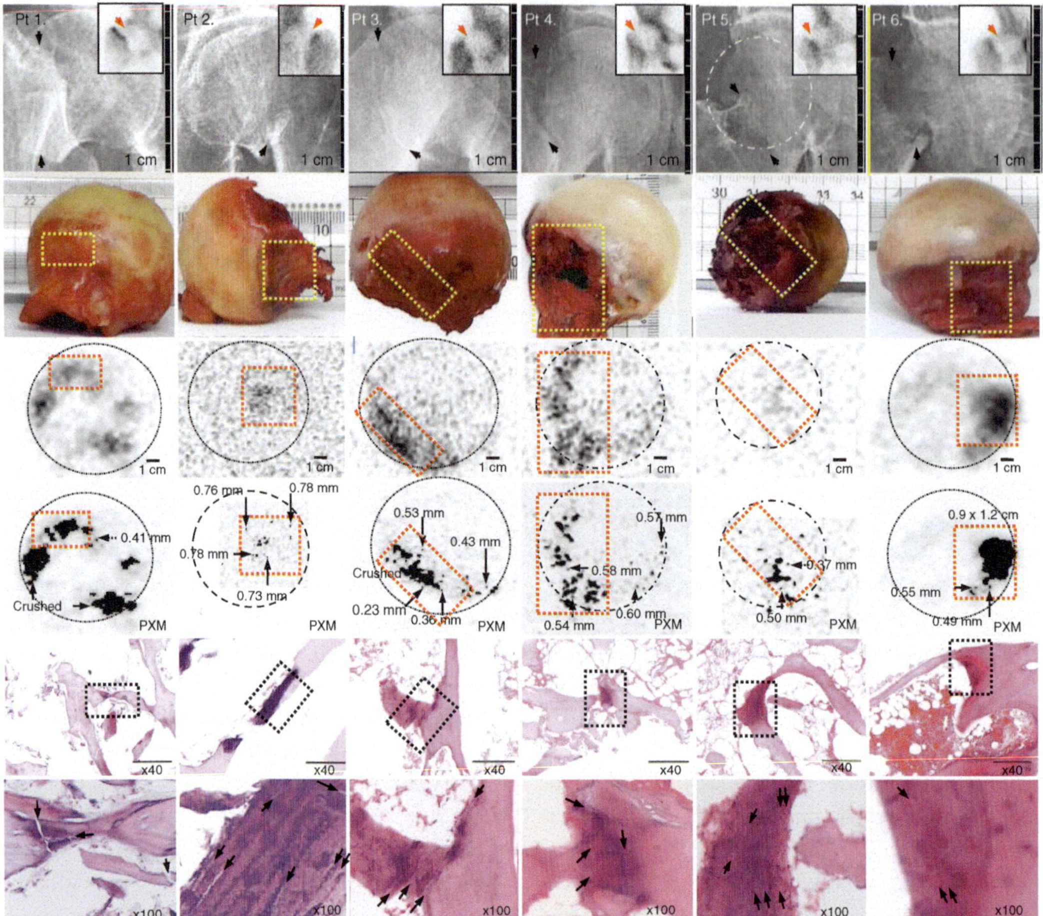

Fig. 14.1 Patients, examinations, and results. Top panel: preoperative anteroposterior radiographs show femoral neck fracture with osteoporosis (*arrowhead*). Inset is preoperative ^{99m}Tc-HDP pinhole bone scan showing avascular photopenia in femoral heads (*red arrows*). Second panel: fresh surgically removed femoral heads show neck fracture with a ruler for basic size measurement and the selection of region of interest (*frame*). Third panel: the naive pinhole scans of specimen show blurry pathological and background ^{99m}Tc-HDP uptake (*frame*). Fourth panel: GCPBS show unsuppressed pinpointed, speckled, geographic, and crushed trabecular fractures. Observe that the tracer uptake in normal and edema and hemorrhage is suppressed. The size microfractures were measured using the pixelized method (PXM; Jung et al. 2016). Fifth panel: the low power view (×40) of H&E stain shows base stain. Patient 6 shows hemorrhage. Bottom panel: the high power H&E stain (×100) shows linear microfractures in all patients. The fractures are well defined in Patients 1—3 and poorly defined in Patients 4—6 (*black arrows*)

gamma correction pinhole bone scan (GCPBS) is useful to specifically image the callused trabecular microfracture (Bahk et al. 2010; Bahk et al. 2016) and most recently it was histopathologically verified in rat experiment (Bahk et al. 2016). It is to be emphatically remarked that ^{99m}Tc-HDP pinhole bone scan is able to uniquely provide bone metabolic profile at the same time.

GCPBS can discern fractured trabeculae from healthy one because the ^{99m}Tc-HDP uptake in fracture is fixed and unsuppressed by gamma correction, whereas the tracer uptake in normal and edema dipped or hemorrhage irritated trabeculae are unfixed and suppressed. In Francis et al. (1980), Francis et al. published an important finding of the fact that high ^{99m}Tc-diphosphonates uptake takes place in acute osteoneogenesis in actively healing fractures in rats. They found that ^{99m}Tc-diphosphonates are more richly adsorbed onto amorphous calcium phosphate, which has more osteogenetic sites than the crystalline hydroxyapatite of normal bone. Furthermore, a recent histobiochemical study confirmed that the morphobiochemical diagnosis of actively calcifying CTMF is possible using ACDSee-10 gamma correction ^{99m}Tc-HDP pinhole bone scan (Bahk et al. 2017).

14.1 Preoperative Diagnosis of Femoral Neck Fracture Using Conventional Radiography and ^{99m}Tc-HDP Pinhole Bone Scan

Preoperatively, the femoral neck fracture with avascular necrosis of the femoral head was confirmed in each patient using conventional radiograph (Fig. 14.1: top panel) and ^{99m}Tc-HDP pinhole scan (Fig. 14.1: top panel inset). The anteroposterior conventional radiograph of the fractured hip joint was taken 24 hours before surgery using an automatic radiographic machine (Siemens Axiom Aristo MX, Erlangen, Germany) and ^{99m}Tc-HDP pinhole bone scan was taken using gamma camera (Siemens E-cam signature, Knoxville, OH, USA). Radiographic exposure factors were 65–70 kVp, 35–40 mAs, and 100-cm source-image distance and the anterior pinhole scan factors were 925–1110 MBq (25–30 mCi) ^{99m}Tc-HDP, 7-min scan time and 12-cm pinhole-aperture-to-object distance, which uniformly covered whole large joints including the shoulder, hip, and knee in adult without distortion. Pinhole aperture size was 4 mm in diameter.

14.2 Gamma Correction ^{99m}Tc-HDP Pinhole Bone Scan of Surgical Specimens and Correlation of Thereof and H&E Stain Findings for Histological Validation

The gamma correction ^{99m}Tc-HDP pinhole bone scans was performed in six consecutive surgical specimens with devascularized femoral heads operatively removed for the arthroplastic treatment of femoral neck fracture (Fig. 14.1 second panel). The age of patients ranged from 72 to 92 years (mean = 78.4) including three males and three females. The fracture involved the right femoral neck in five patients and the left in one patient. The femoral head was removed three to 7 days after fracture. Necrotized femoral head with a portion of the subcapital neck was attained by operation in each patient 24 hours after the diagnostic confirmation of femoral neck fracture with the avascular necrosis of the femoral head. Injuries in the surface of the specimen were first surveyed using a surgical surface microscopy (Fig. 14.1: second panel), imaged using a ^{99m}Tc-HDP pinhole scanner (Fig. 14.1: third panel), and processed using ACDSee-7 gamma correction (Fig. 14.1: fourth panel). Histological diagnosis of each specimen was confirmed by low and high power H&E stain (Fig. 14.1: fifth and sixth panels).

As a representative demonstration of the region of interest, the femoral head specimen of Patient 3 was scrutinized first using a magnifying optic lens (Fig. 14.2a) and then using surgical microscope (OPMI pico, Carl Zeiss, Germany) confirming that seed-pearl-like calluses are already formed (Fig. 14.2b). CTMF was histologically verified (Fig.14.2c) Thereafter, the findings observed were meticulously correlated with those of serial naïve ^{99m}Tc-HDP PBS (Fig. 14.2d) and ACDSee 7 gamma correction pinhole bone scan (Fig. 14.2e) for validation. As anticipated, the gamma correction view showed variously shaped callused micro- and macrotrabecular fractures with unsuppressed high ^{99m}Tc-HDP uptake. The radioactivity so detected was derived from the un-decayed residua of bone tracer intravenously administered to each patient for 24-hour preoperative pinhole bone scanning. The amount of tracer remained, aperture-to-object distance, field of view size, and matrix size were 1.0–1.07 GBq (3.7–4.0 mCi), 12 cm, 14 x 14 cm, and 256 × 256, respectively. Those data were provided for the mathematic size calculation of pixelized microuptake. Photons accumulated ranged from 14 to 23 Kilocounts and the specimen scan time was from 10 to 30 min depending on the amount of residual radioactivity (Bahk et al. 2017).

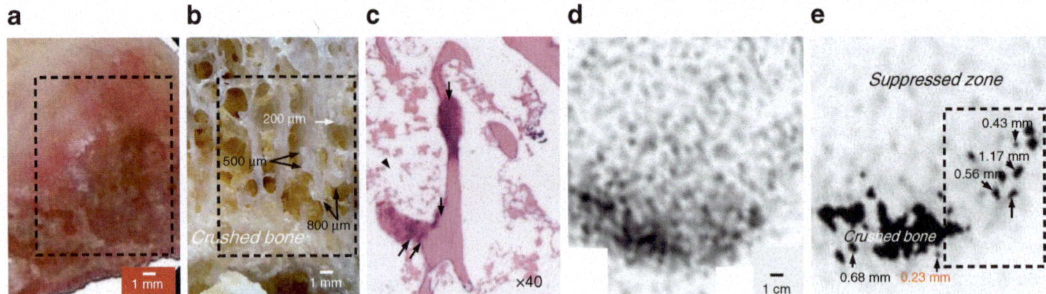

Fig. 14.2 Histopathological validation of callused trabecular microcalluses in femoral neck fracture. (**a**) ×2 magnified low power magnifying lens view of roughened fracture surface shows seed-pearly trabecular changes. (**b**) ×2 magnified surgical microscopic view of broken surface shows callused trabecular microfractures and crushed and normal trabeculae. The smallest microfracture measures 200 µm in size. (**c**) H&E stain shows callused trabecular microfracture with a typical base stain. (**d**) 35°counterclockwise rotated naïve ^{99m}Tc-HDP pinhole bone scan shows nonspecific blurry tracer uptake. The rotation is to match with pathological findings. (**d**) Naïve ^{99m}Tc-HDP pinhole hole bone scan shows nonspecific blurry tracer uptake. (**e**) ACDSee-7 gamma correction view highlights mircocalluses with penumbra (*frame*). The smallest trabecular microfracture measures 0.23 mm or 230 µm in size. The size of microfractures was measured using the pixelized method (PXM; Jung et al. 2016)

14.3 Gamma Correction ^{99m}Tc-HDP Pinhole Bone Scan

Gamma correction (ACDSee-7 version) was performed to radiobiochemically differentiate unfixed ^{99m}Tc-HDP uptake from fixed uptake. The unfixed lower uptake was suppressed, but the fixed higher uptake was not. Methodologically, the original naïve pinhole scan of each specimen (Fig. 14.2d) was processed using gamma correction to discern individual micro ^{99m}Tc-HDP uptake (Fig. 14.2e). The gamma value was increased to suppress the lower tracer uptake in normal and edema and the moderate uptake in hemorrhage is suppressed so that the high chemically bound tracer uptake in CTMF remained unsuppressed and highlighted. Technically, gamma correction was processed by clicking the toolbars in the following sequence (Bahk et al. 2010): Exposure and auto-exposure to maximize uptake intensity and done and save with a new name. Then, exposure and image-brightness control were done by increasing gamma value up to 95 starting from 50 (the default value) and done and save the final image with another new name. The use of an original naïve digital information and communications in medicine (DICOM) was required.

14.4 H&E Stain of Callused Trabecular Microfractures

Each surgical specimen was decalcified and embedded in a paraffin block. The block was cut in 10-µm thickness using a rotary microtome (RM2255, Leica, Germany). The sections were scanned using a virtual microscope (OLIVIA, Olympus, Japan) and treated by hematoxylin-eosin (H&E) stain. For the easier and more accurate comparison of the microfractures shown on gamma correction pinhole bone scan, photomicrograph, and fresh surgical specimen were all twofold magnified (Fig. 14.3).

14.5 Identification of Callused Trabecular Microfracture on ^{99m}Tc-HDP Gamma Correction Pinhole Bone Scan with H&E Stain Validation

Callused trabecular microfracture (CTMF) can be neatly demonstrated and diagnosed using gamma correction pinhole bone scanning (GCPBS) as 99mTc-diphosphonate is specifically adsorbed, fixed, and kept unsuppressed by

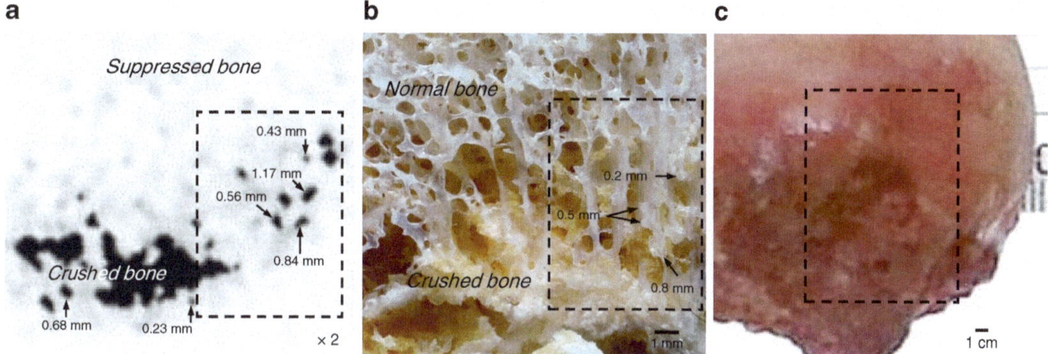

Fig. 14.3 For the more accurate recognition of the microfractures shown on ACDSee-7 gamma correction ^{99m}Tc-HDP pinhole bone scan, photomicrograph, and fresh surgical specimen were twofold magnified. (**a**) The magnified gamma correction pinhole scan view shows highlighted microcalluses (*frame*). The smallest callus measures 0.23 mm (230 μm). (**b**) The magnified surgical microscopic view of the cut surface shows multiple callused microfractures (*frame*), crushed trabeculae, and normal trabeculae. (**c**) Magnified view of the fresh surgical specimen shows the demonstration of blurry seed-pearl-like microfractures (*frame*)

gamma correction (Bahk et al. 2010, 2016). The individual trabecular fractures are imaged as the unsuppressed pinpointed, speckled, round, ovoid, rod-like, archipelagic, and geographic high uptake (Fig. 14.3a) as verified by H&E staining which is carried out in two steps. The first step is to find the region of interest using a low power view (Fig. 14.1. fifth panel) and the second step is to identify the calcifying CTMF stained in the base to surround whitish thready microfractures in high power H&E stain (Fig. 14.1. bottom panel). The reciprocal correlation of the findings of GCPBS and H&E stain rendered us to confirm that the calcifying calluses are actively formed in trabecular fractures.

14.6 Quantification of Unsuppressed ^{99m}Tc-HDP Uptake in Callused Trabecular Microfracture by Pixelized Measurement

The size of the individual micro ^{99m}Tc-HDP uptake in trabecular microfracture was mathematically calculated using the pixelized measurement method (Yoon et al. 2015; Jung et al. 2016) or using a magnifying lens (vide infra). Each individual microspot was appointed as a region of interest. The image profile is presented in a line spread function denoting the signal intensity of the applied line. The y-axis of image profile is the signal intensity and the x-axis shows the pixel number in profile. In order to easily measure the full width at half maximum matrix size was expanded to 512 × 512. Because of the increased number of pixels, the signal intensity value was assigned by interpolation at the expanded bin which does not have a signal intensity value. To interpolate the between bins, the Gaussian curve fitting method was used using the in-house MATLAB code (Mathworks, R 2011a, USA) [20]. The equation of the Gaussian curve fitting was as below:

$$y(x) = \frac{1}{\sigma\sqrt{2\pi}} \exp\left[-\frac{(x - x_0)^2}{2\sigma^2}\right]$$

y = interpolated value
x = original frame value
x_0 = mean value of the frame value
σ = standard deviation

14.6.1 Statistical Analysis

We measured the intensity of ^{99m}Tc-HDP uptake using the NIH ImageJ densitometry in the seriated naïve PBS and GCPBS in 10 consecutive patients. The lowest ^{99m}Tc-HDP uptake intensity was 10.8 AU in a normal trabeculae and the highest uptake intensity was 243.2 AU in a microfracture. All measured data were statistically analyzed using the GraphPad Prism (n.d.) (San Diago, USA). As shown in detail in Table 14.1, difference was significant between normal and edema (P value ≤ 0.001) and higher significance were noted among edema, hemorrhage, and microfracture (P value <0.0001) (Bahk et al. 2019).

14.6.2 Magnifying Optic Lens Measurement of Callused Trabecular Microfracture

Callused trabecular microfracture (CTMF) can also be directly measured using an ordinary optic magnifying lens in terms of pixel. This method is simple and easy to perform as far as the image is sharply defined without penumbra as provided by ACDSee-10 gamma correction (Fig. 14.4).

Table 14.1 Ninety five (95) sampled data were statistically treated using the GraphPad Prism (n.d.) (San Diago, U.S.A.). Results were highly significant (∗∗ P-value was less than 0.001 and ∗∗∗ P-value was less than 0.000.1), respectively. Also shows NIH Arbitrary Unit with a standard deviation of normal, edematous, hemorrhagic, and fractured trabeculae

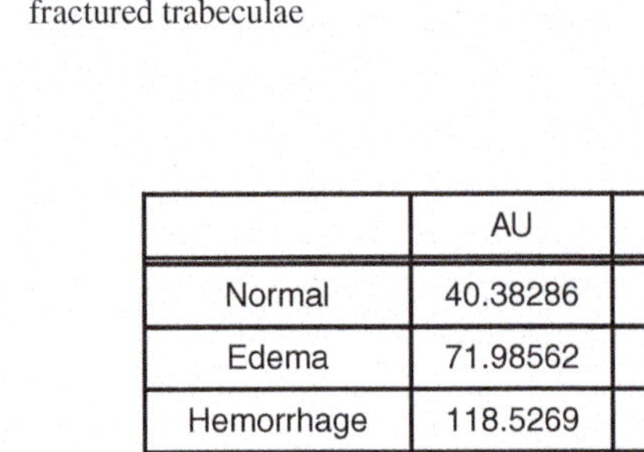

	AU	SD
Normal	40.38286	5.12296
Edema	71.98562	7.792942
Hemorrhage	118.5269	13.52758
Fracture	198.8583	33.94485

AU = artbitray unit and SD = standard deviation.
** P value : < 0.001
*** P value : < 0.0001

Fig. 14.4 Callused trabecular microfracture can be directly measured using an ordinary optic magnifying lens in terms of pixel. This method is simple and easy to perform as far as the image is sharply defined without penumbra which is provided by ACDSee-10 version of gamma correction. ACDSee-7 version suffers from penumbra making measurement to rely on mathematic calculation (Fig. 13.1b). (**a**) The resected specimen surface, cleansed by 10% formaldehyde solution, was scrutinized using surface microscope that shows seed-pearly callused trabecular microfractures. The smallest one measures 0.2 mm in size. (**b**) Gamma correction pinhole scan shows callused trabecular microfractures with the smallest ones measuring 200 um in size. (**c**) 10× magnifying lens. (**d**) Unit pixel measures 200 μm in size

It is to be noted that ACDSee-7 suffers from penumbra (Fig. 13.1b).

14.7 Overall Considerations

The characteristics of patients were presented in Fig. 14.1. Six patients consisted of 3 males and 3 females with the age ranging from 72 to 92 years and a mean was 78.4 years. The causes of femoral neck fracture were falling down from bed or chair, staircase, or tumbling in washroom or street. The imaging diagnosis of femoral neck fracture was made in each patient: first and anatomically using plain radiography (Fig. 14.1: top panel proper) and second and radiobiochemically using ^{99m}Tc-HDP pinhole bone scanning (Fig. 14.1: top panel inset). On the day next, the devascularized femoral head with a portion of the subcapital neck was removed by surgery to perform arthroplasty (Fig. 14.1: second panel). Femoral head specimens were checked immediately after surgical operation using a reading glass (Fig. 14.1: second panel) and imaged using pinhole scanner (Fig. 14.1: third panel) and the scanned image was processed using gamma correction to demonstrate TMF (Fig. 14.1: fourth panel). Subsequently, the injured surface of specimens was cleansed using 10% formalin solution and scrutinized using surgical surface microscope to confirm the formation of microfractures (Fig. 14.2b), and lastly, the CTMF were reciprocally inter-correlated among the findings of surgical specimen, surface microscopy, H&E stain GCPBS, and serial naïve and gamma correction pinhole scans (Fig. 14.2). Histolopathologically, CTMF was shown as a whitish thready shadow within purple basophilic stained matrix. Their numbers were plural and shapes were either sharply or poorly defined (Fig. 14.1: bottom panel).

The naïve pinhole scan of the specimens showed irregular areas of blurry ^{99m}Tc-HDP uptake of various intensities obscuring fracture (Fig. 14.1: third panel). However, the post-gamma correction view distinctly highlighted variously shaped CTMF with unsuppressed high tracer uptake (Fig. 14.1: fourth panel). The shape was pinpointed, speckled, rod-like, and geographic or crushed. Crushed fractures occasionally contained lucent microdefects. This finding proves the fineness of gamma correction image resolution. For quantitation, the size of individual microfractures was calculated using pixelized measurement (Fig.14.2e) (Jung et al. 2016). The smallest microfracture in each of six patients was 0.41 mm, 0.73 mm, 0.23 mm, 0.54 mm, 0.37 mm, and 0.49 mm (mean = 0.46 mm), respectively. Of these, the smallest microfracture of 0.23 mm occurred in patient 3 in this series (Fig. 14.1: fourth panel). There were large crushed fractures with unwashed ^{99m}Tc-HDP uptake in patients 1, 3, and 6. Fractures were sharply defined in patients 1, 2, and 3 and un-sharply defined in patients 4, 5, and 6. The difference was not related to posttraumatic duration and was considered to be due to the different physical impact of trauma and the unequal nature and degree of callus formation. The surgical microscopic findings of seed-pearly microfractures and crushed bone in patient 3 (Fig. 14.3e) were in good accord with the pinpointed and crushed bone ^{99m}Tc-HDP uptake in GCPBS and moderate accord was observed in all other patients. Low power H&E stain view showed basophilic injured trabeculae in the bone marrow space with probable edematous effacement (patients 1 and 2), dominant fat cell infiltration and fibrosis (patients 3–5), and overt hemorrhage (patient 6). In contrast, x100 view showed a distinctly visualized fine fracture in patients 1–3 and mere typical base stain in the remainder.

Generally, the scrutiny and correlation of findings shown in surgical specimen, GCPBS, surgical microscope, and H&E stain were in good accord individually and altogether, proving that they are trabecular microfractures (Figs. 14.1, 14.2, and 14.3). To be detailed, for example, in Patient 3, the preoperative conventional radiograph with a therein insetted pinhole bone scan, resected surgical specimen and its naïve and gamma correction ^{99m}Tc-HDP pinhole scans, surgical microscopy, and H&E stain confirmed the femoral neck fracture, femoral head surface injuries, hazy ^{99m}Tc-HDP uptake, and distinct pathological micro uptake, seed-pearly microcal-

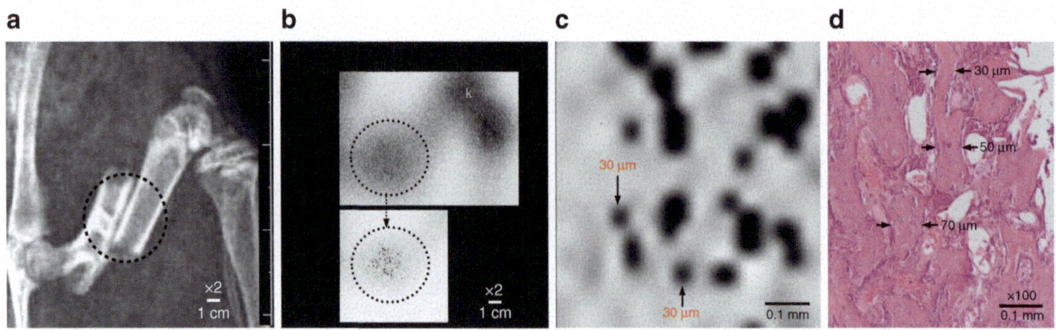

Fig. 14.5 Normal control 30-week-old young rat. ×2 enlarged view. (**a**) Radiograph shows a fracture in the mid-shaft of the femur with marked contraction deformity and 1-cm scale (*ring*). The knee shows actively growing physes. (**b**) Top frame: naïve ^{99m}Tc-HDP animal pinhole scan shows blurry tracer uptake (*frame*) with physiological tracer uptake in growing knee bones (*k*) and bottom frame shows post-suppression tracer uptake in microfracture. (**c**) ×100 enlarged view. (**d**) H&E stain shows variously sized trabecular microfractures with endosteal rimming and diffuse marrow hemorrhage

lus formation, and thready and meshy fractures with basophilic H&E stain (Fig.14.2). All these findings present actively calcifying trabecular fractures. Conclusively, GCPBS can finely image the callused trabecular microfracture with pinpointed, speckled, rod-like, and geometric ^{99m}Tc-HDP uptake and also crushed trabeculae. Furthermore, GCPBS can distinguish actively calcifying microfracture with unsuppressed ^{99m}Tc-HDP uptake from edema and hemorrhage dipped trabeculae with suppressed tracer uptake as far as trabeculae is not injured.

Trabecular microfracture ubiquitously occurs in almost all bone diseases (Vernon-Roberts and Pirie 1973; Mandalia and Henson 2008; McFarland PH and Frost 1973; Bahk 2013; Fazzalari 1993) and also even in normal physiological activity and daily works (Frost 1973; Tassani and Matsopoulos 2013). Trabecular microfracture is nothing but the simple breakage of trabeculae which measures approx. 0.5 mm in thickness (Vernon-Roberts B and Pirie CJ) and heals by callus formation. The callus is a micronodular aggregate of woven bone and it is seed-pearl like in appearance (Fig. 14.3). Clinically, GCPBS can be used for the diagnosis of occult fractures (Bahk et al. 2010) and other bone diseases (Bahk 2013). Contusion may incite trabecular microfracture and/or endoblastic rimming which can be precisely diagnosed using the ^{99m}Tc-HDP gamma correction pinhole bone scan. The endosteal rimming reaction to trabecular injury was experimentally produced and confirmed in young rats (Fig. 14.4) (Bahk et al. 2016). In addition, the imaging differentiation of bone marrow edema, bone marrow hemorrhage, and CTMF was also published most lately (Fig. 14.5) (Bahk et al. 2019) (vide infra). All those studies were performed using a gamma correction pinhole bone scan. Gamma correction ^{99m}Tc-HDP pinhole bone scan can distinguish the intact trabeculae with suppressible meager tracer uptake from injured trabeculae with un-suppressible tracer uptake (Fig. 14.6). Such differential ^{99m}Tc-HDP uptake is considered to be highly helpful for the specific distinction of bone edema, bone hemorrhage, and trabecular microfracture as it will be fully discussed in the following chapter.

A review of literature revealed interesting publications on this theme reflecting increasing medical concern on the imaging diagnosis of trabecular microfracture. They are micro-CT (Okazaki et al. 2014), multi-slice cone-beam CT (Klintstrom et al. 2014), and the micro-MRI (Song and Wehrli 1999; Rajapakse et al. 2012). Gamma correction ^{99m}Tc-HDP pinhole bone scan is another efficient, convenient, and economical means to specifically diagnose callused trabecular microfracture using simple ^{99m}Tc-HDP pinhole bone scanning.

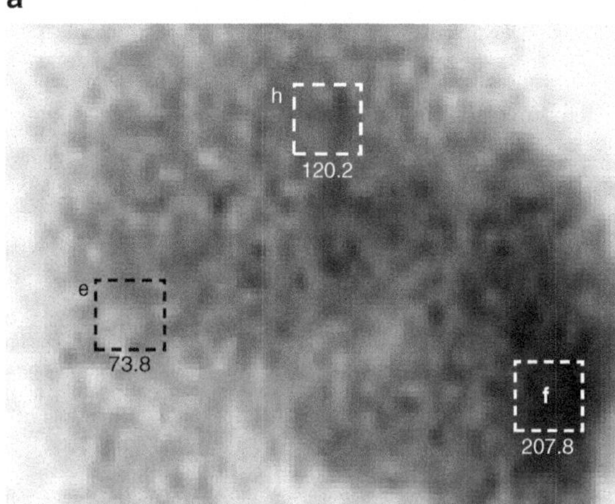

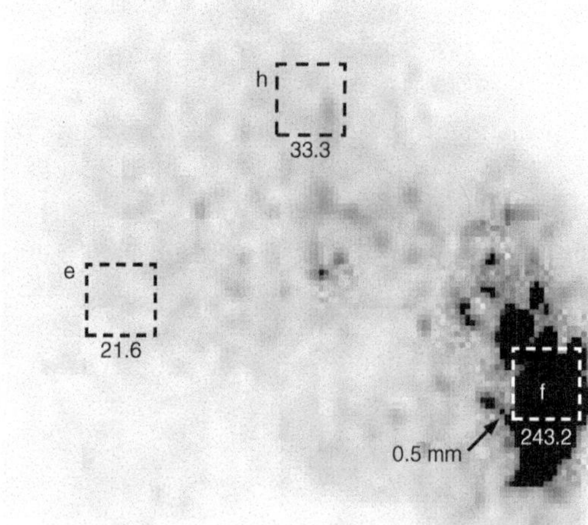

Fig. 14.6 Edema and hemorrhage can be differentiated using GCPBS and NIH's ImageJ densitometry. The figure presents the suppressed ^{99m}Tc-HDP uptake feature of edema and hemorrhage and highlighted tracer uptake in fractures. (**a**) Naïve pinhole scan shows three 1-cm^2 areas of blurry tracer uptake of edema (*e*) and hemorrhage (*h*) and fracture (*f*) with AU values: the uptake in edema is 73.8, in hemorrhage is 120.2 and in fracture is 207.8. (**b**) Gamma correction suppresses edema and hemorrhage uptake highlighting fractures (*f*) with an increased value of AU. The smallest fracture measures 500 μm in size. A large ovoid fracture is marked with f. Increased AU value in fracture after comma correction is due to enhanced signal-to-noise ratio

This ^{99m}Tc-HDP pinhole bone scan imaging and histological study was prospectively performed for two aims using surgically removed specimens of traumatically devascularized femoral head recruited from *six* consecutive patients. The first aim was to histologically validate that GCPBS can demonstrate the actively forming callused trabecular microfracture and the second was to biochemically confirm the differential suppression of ^{99m}Tc-HDP uptake between edema and hemorrhage and callused microfracture. The results showed that gamma correction can cleanly suppress the low ^{99m}Tc-HDP uptake in normal bone and also the mild and moderate uptake in edematous and hemorrhagic trabeculae (Fig. 14.5).

The size of the callused trabecular microfracture was measured using pixelized method (Yoon et al. 2014, 2015; Jung et al. 2016). Actually, the size was calculated by measuring the FWHM of the signal peak. The results of our gamma correction study showed that the pinpoint and otherwise shaped ^{99m}Tc-HDP uptake shown on the surgical surface micrograph (Fig. 14.3e) and GCPBS (Fig. 14.3f) was in good accord, attesting to the fact that the micro ^{99m}Tc-HDP uptake denotes microfractures. Furthermore, the multifactorial intercorrelation of the findings of GCPBS, surgical microscope, and H&E stain all showed generalized good accord in morphology (Fig. 14.2).

In order to image trabecular microfractures, synchrotron radiation micro CT was used obtaining a 3D image of the microfracture in osteoporotic femoral head as we did in this experiment. Our study was exclusively focused on the individual callused trabecular microfracture imaged with unsuppressed high ^{99m}Tc-HDP uptake. The trabecular size ranged from 0.23 to 0.54 mm ($n = 6$; mean = 0.46 mm). It is to be noted that our gamma correction pinhole bone scan study is specifically limited to trabecular mirofractures, whereas the synchrotron radiation micro-CT images callus and trabeculae as a unit causing image aberration. Strong radiobiochemical advantage of GCPBS is that it can uniquely provide the information on bone metabolic profile in callused trabecular microfractures enabling us to assess the healing of the trabecular microfracture in qualitative and quantitative manners when clinically desired.

In conclusion, GCPBS can simultaneously make fine morphological and biochemical diagnosis of actively healing callused trabecular microfracture at the level of 230 um in size. It can also distinguish the callused trabecular microfractures with characteristically unsuppressed high ^{99m}Tc-HDP uptake from intact and edematous or hemorrhagic trabeculae with suppressible tracer uptake. GCPBS is easy to perform and economical providing us with useful morphological and biochemical information on callused trabecular microfracture.

References

Bahk YW. Gamma correction pinhole bone scan diagnosis. In: Bahk YW, editor. Combined scintigraphic and radiographic diagnosis of bone and joint diseases: including gamma correction interpretation. 4th ed. Berlin: Springer Verlag; 2013. p. 209–89.

Bahk YW, Jeon HS, Kim JM, et al. Novel use of gamma correction for precise ^{99m}Tc-HDP pinhole bone scan diagnosis and classification of knee occult fracture. Skeletal Radiol. 2010;39:807–13.

Bahk YW, Chung YA, Lee WY, et al. Gamma correction ^{99m}Tc-hydroxy methylene diphosphonate pinhole bone scan diagnosis and histopathological verification of trabecular contusion in young rats. Nucl Med Commun. 2016;37:986–91.

Bahk YW, Hwang SH, Lee UY, et al. Morphobiochemical diagnosis of acute trabecular microfractures using gamma correction Tc-99m HDP pinhole bone scan with histopathological verification. Medicine®. 2017;96(45):e8419.

Bahk YW, Kim EE, Chung YA, et al. Precise differential diagnosis of acute bone marrow edema and hemorrhage and trabecular microfractures using naïve and gamma correction pinhole bone scans. J Internat Med Research. 2019; https://doi.org/10.1177/0300060518819910.

Fazzalari NL. Trabecular microfracture. Calcif Tissue Int. 1993;53(Suppl 1):S143. Discussion S6–7.

Francis MD, Ferguson DL, Tofe AJ, Bevan JA, Michaels SE. Comparative evaluation of three diphosphonates: in vitro adsorption (C- 14 labeled) and in vivo osteogenic uptake (Tc-99m complexed). J Nucl Med. 1980;21:1185–9.

Frost HM. The spinal osteoporoses. Mechanisms of pathogenesis and pathophysiology. Clin Endocrinol Metab. 1973;2:257–75.

Jung JY, Cheon GJ, Lee YS, Ha S, et al. Pixelized measurement of ^{99m}Tc-HDP micro particles formed in gamma correction phantom pinhole scan: a reference study. Nucl Med Mol Imaging. 2016;50:207–2212.

Klintstrom E, Smedby O, Moreno R, Brismar TB. Trabecular bone structure parameters from 3D image processing of clinical multi-slice and cone-beam computed tomography data. Skelet Radiol. 2014;43:197–204.

Mandalia V, Henson JH. Traumatic bone bruising: a review article. Eur J Radiol. 2008;67:54–61.

McFarland PH, Frost HL. A possible cause for aseptic necrosis of the femoral head. Henry Ford Med Bull. 1961;9:115–22.

Mink JH, Deutsch AL. Occult cartilage and bone injuries of the knee: detection, nee: histology and cryosections in 5 cases. Acta Orthop Scand. 1989;69:291–4.

Okazaki N, Chiba K, Taguchi K, Nango N, Kubota S, Ito M, et al. Trabecular microfractures in the femoral head with osteoporosis: analysis of microcallus formations by synchrotron radiation micro CT. Bone. 2014;64:82–7.

Rajapakse CS, Leonard MB, Bhagat YA, Sun W, Magland JF, Wehrli FW. Micro-MR imaging-based computational biomechanics demonstrates reduction in cortical and trabecular bone strength after renal transplantation. Radiology. 2012;262:912–20.

Rangger C, Kathrein A, Freund MC, et al. Bone bruise of the knee: histology and cryosections in 5 cases. Acta Orthop Scand. 1998;69:291–4.

Ryu KN, Jin W, Ko YT, Yoon Y, Oh JH, Park YK, et al. Bone bruises: MR characteristics and histological correlation in the young pig. Clin Imaging. 2000;24:371–80.

Song HK, Wehrli FW. In-vivo micro-imaging using alternating navigator echoes with applications to cancellous bone structural analysis. Magn Reson Med. 1999;41:947–53.

Tassani S, Matsopoulos GK. The micro-structure of bone trabecular fracture: an inter-site study. Bone. 2013;60:78–86.

Vernon-Roberts B, Pirie CJ. Healing trabecular microfractures in the bodies of lumbar vertebrae. Ann Rheum Dis. 1973;32:406–12.

Yao L, Lee JK. Occult intraosseous fracture: detection with MR imaging. Radiology. 1988;167:749–51.

Yoon DK, Jung JY, Hong KJ, Suh TS. Tomographic image of prompt gamma ray from boron neutron capture therapy: a Monte Carlo simulation study. Appl Phys Lett. 2014;104:083521.

Yoon DK, Jung JY, Han SM, et al. Statistical analysis for discrimination of prompt gamma ray peak induced by high energy neutron: monte Carlo simulation study. J Radioanal Nucl Chem. 2015;303:859–66.

15 Differential Diagnosis of Bone Marrow Edema and Hemorrhage and Callused Trabecular Microfracture with Gamma Correction ^{99m}Tc-HDP Pinhole Bone Scan Validation

Bone marrow edema (BME), bone marrow hemorrhage (BMH), and trabecular microfracture (TMF) comprise a basic triad of bone marrow pathologies ubiquitously incited by trauma, sports, osteoporosis, inflammation, infection, neoplasm, and even daily physical activities (Salcianu et al. 2014). With the latest development of gamma correction pinhole bone scan (GCPBS) the triad became to be specifically diagnosed in detail using imaging methods, gamma correction ^{99m}TC-HDP pinhole bone scanning in particular (Bahk et al. 2016; Bahk and Chung 2017; Bahk et al. 2017). Such developments more than naturally required there to fit quantitation method to accomplish a precise, systemic diagnosis of BME, BMH, and callused trabecular microfracture (CTMF). Thus, a visuospatial and mathematic assay (VSMA) was worked out to specifically image, distinguish, and measure BME, BMH, and TMF by the integrated use of naïve and ACDSee-7 gamma correction ^{99m}Tc-HDP pinhole bone scans, the NIH ImageJ densitometry, and pixelized size measurement. As mentioned above TMF, BME, and BMF are the triad of the most basic bone marrow changes occurring in nearly all bone diseases. BME is the accumulation of clear serous fluid in bone marrow, BMH is the accumulation of extravasated blood, and CTMF is callused trabecular pathology. Mere BME does not injure trabeculae (Fig. 15.1 top panel), but BMH may well additively hurt already injured trabeculae through the phagocytic actions of neutrophil and monocyte and some other blood ingredients (Fig. 15.1 bottom panel). This investigation was focused on the differentiation of acute BME and BMH as well as TMF. Using the Arbitrary Unit (AU) system of the NIH ImageJ densitometry, http://rsb.info.nih.gov/ij, we were able to sort ^{99m}Tc-HDP uptake into four categories. Normal trabeculae was allocated to be ≤50 AU, edema to be from 51 to 100 AU, hemorrhage to be from 101 to 150 AU, and TMF to be ≥151.

Our earlier GCPBS-histopathological study in young rats showed acute bone contusion to incite the endosteal rimming with unsuppressed high ^{99m}Tc-HDP uptake in trabeculae (Fig. 15.1 bottom panel) (Bahk et al. 2016) and the successive study performed in the surgical specimens of the fractured femoral neck in six consecutive patients showed that fracture incites unsuppressed high ^{99m}Tc-HDP uptake in the callused trabecular microfractures (Fig. 15.2) (Bahk et al. 2017).

The review of literature revealed that a dog model study proved that hemorrhage transforms fatty marrow to become a bone-forming tissue (Yamamura 1994) and a bovine study confirmed hemorrhage to incite change in the shear strength of cement-bone interface (Majkowski et al. 1994). Years later, an arthroscopic study showed trabecular fractures to be linked with hemorrhage in fatty bone marrow (Rangger et al. 1998). The results of all those earlier workers and our own recent GCPBS-histopathological study proved

Y.-W. Bahk, *Imaging of Trabecular Microfracture and Bone Marrow Edema and Hemorrhage*,
https://doi.org/10.1007/978-981-15-4466-8_15

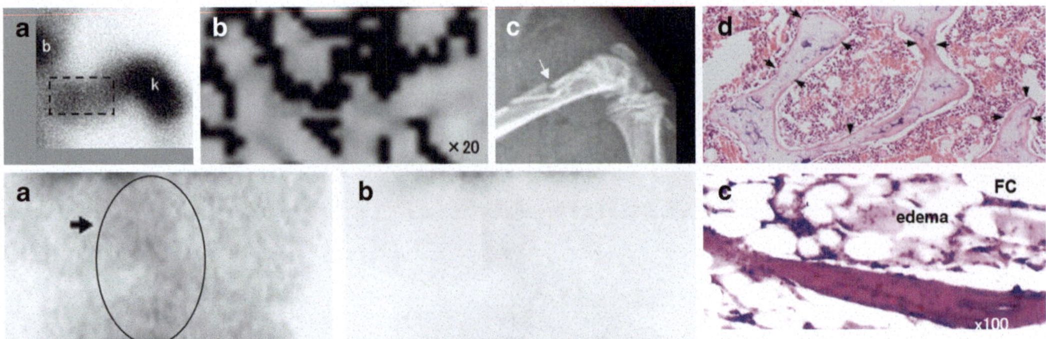

Fig. 15.1 Gamma correction can distinguish fracture from edema and hemorrhage. Top panel: (**a**) Naïve pinhole bone scan shows injured area (*frame*). b is the urinary bladder and *k* is the knee. (**b**) Gamma correction view shows enhanced tracer uptake in endosteal rimming. (**c**) Young rat radiograph shows fracture (*arrow*). (**d**) H&E stain shows typical endosteal rimming with hemorrhage. Bottom panel: (**a**) Naïve pinhole scan of bones the right knee in a 16-year-old male student shows faint edema uptake due to sport injury (*ring* and *arrow*). (**b**) Gamma correction view shows clean suppression of edema. (**c**) H&E stain shows edema and fat cells with intact trabecula, FC is fat cell (from teaching file)

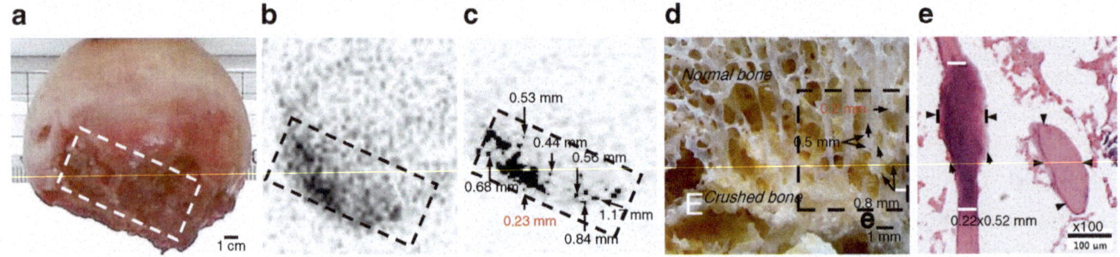

Fig. 15.2 Histological verification of unsuppressed tracer uptake in osteoporotic trabecular microfractures in femoral head in a 72-year-old female. Femoral head was removed for prosthesis. (**a**) Surgical specimen shows roughened fracture surface with seed-pearly trabecular microfractures (*frame*). (**b**) Naïve ^{99m}Tc-HDP pinhole scan shows nonspecific blurry tracer uptake (*frame*). (**c**) Seriated gamma correction view shows suppressed blurry tracer uptake highlighting microfractures. Sizes were measured using pixelized method. Smallest callus was 0.23 mm. (**d**) Surgical microscope of sectioned specimen shows several pearl-seed callused microfractures. The smallest one measures 0.23 mm in size. (**e**) H&E stain shows base stained 0.22 × 0.52 mm microfracture (*arrowheads*) with fine linear and meshy fractures (*arrow*) and endosteal rimming in a trabecula (*arrowheads*)

that simulated and actual hemorrhage can injure trabeculae to incite osteoneogenesis in the form of endosteal rimming and/or seed-pearly callused trabecular microfracture. Theoretically, the callus formed in TMF is considered to be related to the additive injurious effect of hemorrhage to already injured trabeculae which were made vulnerable to hemorrhage. It is radiobiochemically and ^{99m}Tc-HDP pinhole bone scintigraphically interpreted that the highlighted ^{99m}Tc-HDP uptake in acute TMF is due to the avid biochemical incorporation of bone tracer into the amorphous calcium phosphate in injured bone and contrastingly the suppressed uptake in BME and BMH can be ascribed to the mere ^{99m}Tc-HDP adhesion of tracer to crystalline hydroxyapatite (Francis et al. 1980; Salcianu et al. 2014). Clinically, MRI is widely used for the study of BME (Rosenson et al. 1996; Eustace et al. 2001; Korompilias et al. 2009; Thiryayi et al. 2008) but rather limitedly for BMH (Zanetti et al. 2000; Mink and Deutch 1989). Such an unequal biased study is considered to be due to the technical difficulty of specific MR imaging of BMH and its interpretation. In this regard, it was an interesting academic interest that the histopathology–MRI correlation study published by Zanetti et al. showed only "edemalike" change unreferring to hemorrhage despite the presence of small bleeding areas in their chronic arthritis-related bone marrow disease case. Interestingly, the application of gamma correction to Zanetti's MR image showed that "edemalike" change to consist of BME, BMH, and TMF (Fig. 15.3). This retrograde analysis was performed with generous permission of Professor Marco Zanetti and Radiology journal.

Imaging diagnostically, BME, BMH, and TMF can be differentiated from each other using the VSMA (visiospatial mathematic assay; Bahk et al. 2017). This method rendered us to distinguish and categorize four different types of ^{99m}Tc-HDP uptake patterns of BME, BMF, TMF, and normal trabeculae. The lowest uptake of 0.8 AU was observed in normal trabecula and the highest uptake of 243.2 AU in TMF. VSMA is useful to morphologically and quantitatively distinguish BME, BMH, and TMF (Fig. 15.4). In particular, BME can be visually and uptake-value-wise

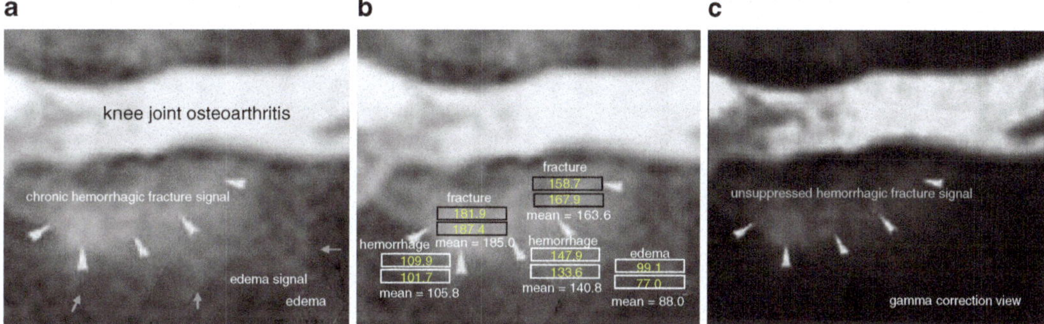

Fig. 15.3 ImageJ densitometry of MR signal intensity in histologically proven "edemalike" change in knee (Zanetti et al. 2000) appears to distinguish edema signal from hemorrhagic fracture signal. This was subchondral bone changes incited by chronic knee joint osteoarthritis. (**a**) Sagittal STIR MR image (4800/30) shows bright signal intensity in chronic hemorrhagic fracture (*arrowhead*). The area defined by arrowheads is hemorrhagic compressed trabeculae. "Edemalike" lesion is presented with lower bright signal intensity (*arrows*). (**b**) Mean values of NIH ImageJ intensity are 88.0 in edema area, 105.8 and 140.8 in hemorrhagic areas, and 185.0 and 163.6 in two trabecular fractures. (**c**) Gamma correction (gamma = 22) MRI shows bright signal intensity in fractures with edema and hemorrhage suppressed out. MR image was used with permissions of Professor Marco Zanetti and Radiology journal

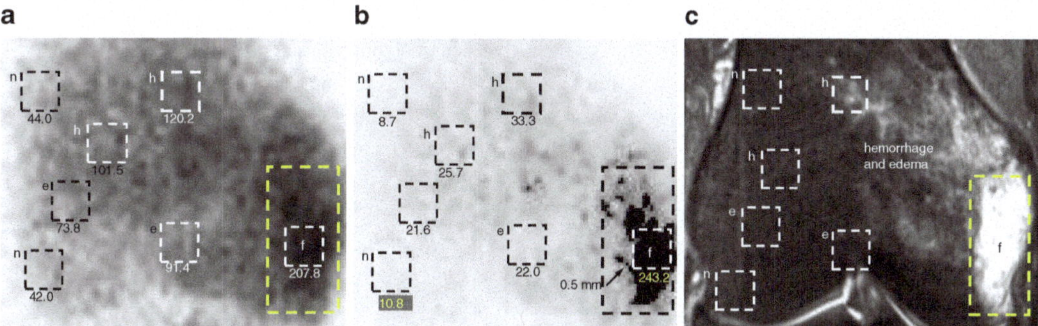

Fig. 15.4 Drifting edema and hemorrhage in cometary fracture involving the left lateral femoral condyle in a 71-year-old male. (**a**) Naïve PBS shows blurry mild and moderate tracer uptake in edema (*e*) and hemorrhage (*h*) (*1-cm² frame*) and intense tracer uptake in fracture (*yellow frame*). There are two areas each of edema, hemorrhage, and normal, and one fracture. Uptake value is 50 or less in normal site, 51–100 in edema, 101–150 in hemorrhage, and 151 or more in fracture. (**b**) Gamma correction suppresses uptake in edema, hemorrhage, and normal trabecula and enhances uptake in fracture. Smallest fracture is 0.5 mm in size and the lowermost AU value is 10.8 in normal trabecula and highest AU is 243.2 in fracture. (**c**) Corroborative coronal FS T2 weighted MR image shows a large ovoid fracture with bright signal intensity (*yellow frame*) and two 1-cm² unit areas each of edema and hemorrhage with less bright signal intensities (*white frames*)

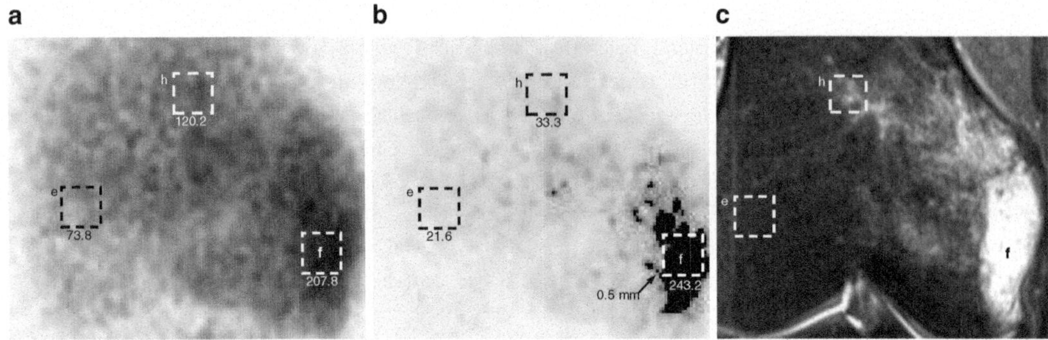

Fig. 15.5 Edema and hemorrhage can be differentiated using GCPBS and ImageJ densitometry. This is an utmost simplified view of Fig. 2 to typically feature suppressed tracer uptake in edema and hemorrhage and highlighted uptake in fractures. (**a**) Naïve pinhole scan shows three 1-cm^2 areas of blurry tracer uptake of edema (*e*) and hemorrhage (*h*) and fracture (*f*) with AU values: Edema uptake 73.8, hemorrhage uptake 120.2 and fracture 207.8. (**b**) Gamma correction suppresses edema and hemorrhage uptake clearly highlighting fractures (*f*). Smallest fracture measured 0.5 mm. (**c**) Corroborative FS coronal T2-weighted MR image (3500/18) shows a 1-cm^2 area of hemorrhage (*h*) with bright signal intensity and another 1-cm^2 area of edema with mild bright signal intensity (*e*). A large ovoid fracture is marked with f

distinguished from BMH. ^{99m}Tc-HDP uptake was mild in edema and moderate in hemorrhage and the difference was objectively calculated using the NIH ImageJ densitometry, for example, 73.8 AU in edema and 120.2 AU in hemorrhage (Fig. 15.5).

We used the AU classification of ImageJ densitometry in this study based on three rationales. First, TMF was distinguished as such using GCPBS image (Fig. 15.5). Second, the NIH ImageJ densitometry permitted easy and precise measurement of different ^{99m}Tc-HDP uptake in seriated naïve and gamma correction pinhole bone scans. Third, the injurious effect of the higher viscous hemorrhaged blood was considered to be stronger than that of the lower viscous edema. Actually, the viscosity of edema is 1.27 ± 0.06 mPa.s and blood is 3.26 ± 0.43 mPa.s (Rosenson et al. 1996) and the latter contains neutrophils and monocyte that yield phagocytic action by nature (Williams et al. Gray's Anatomy). It is of interest that a mathematic model of bone fracture healing was published by Pivonka and Dunstan (2012). Their model consists of four phases including an initial inflammatory phase, two repair phases with soft callus formation and hard callus formation, and finally physiological remodeling phase. The data they attained indicated that environmental conditions such as blood supply and the availability of mesenchymal stem cells are crucial for fracture healing. In this connection, we were convinced that the precise imaging of BME, BMH, and TMF and the regular quantitation of bone metabolic change, for example, in terms of AU, significantly contribute to the advancement of the diagnosis and treatment of MBE, BMH, and TMF.

In conclusion, BME, BMH, and TMF can now be finely imaged and differentially diagnosed using VSMA that technically consists of seriated naïve PBS-and-GCPBS assessment, the NIH ImageJ uptake intensity densitometry, and pixelized measurement. VSMA can distinguish BME from BMH and distinctly demonstrate TMF. Radiobiochemically, the ^{99m}Tc-HDP uptake in normal trabecula, BME, and BMH was suppressed by gamma correction, but the tracer uptake in TMF was contrarily enhanced distinctly highlighting its presence. The uptake intensities are 50 AU or less in normal site, 51–100 AU in BME, 101–150 AU in BMH, and 151 or more AU in TMF. The smallest TMF in our series was 230 μm and the lowest post-gamma correction tracer uptake was 10.8 AU in intact trabecula and the highest tracer uptake was 243.2 AU in TMF.

Incidentally but importantly, the harmlessness of edema to normal trabeculae can be verified using VSMA. Actually as shown in Fig. 15.6 a

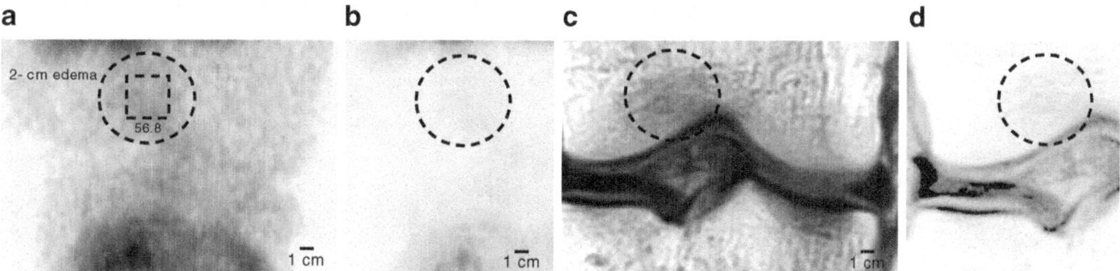

Fig. 15.6 Innocuousness of edema to trabeculae. This smallest edema seen in our series occurred in the right femoral intercondylar fossa was due to motor vehicle accident in a 16-year-old male student (*circle*). (**a**) Naïve ^{99m}Tc-HDP pinhole bone scan shows 2-cm edema. Tracer uptake value in 1-cm unit area measured using ImageJ densitometry was 56.8, a near lowest value of edema (*circle*). (**b**) Gamma correction view shows the suppression of tracer uptake (*circle*). (**c**) Corroborative coronal T1-weighted (460/26) MR image shows edema with dark signal intensity (*circle*). (**d**) Gamma correction MR image shows suppression of dark signal MR intensity of edema with no architectural change (*circle*)

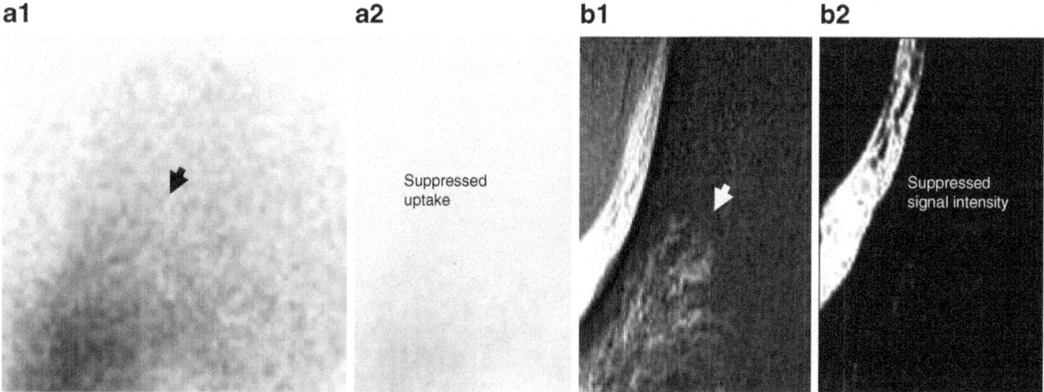

Fig. 15.7 Suppression of a large fan-shaped bone marrow edema in the left medial femoral condyle incited by motor vehicle contusion in a 24-year-old male. (**a1**) Naïve ^{99m}Tc-HDP pinhole scan shows a large edema with increased tracer uptake (*arrow*). (**a2**) Gamma correction view shows neat suppression of the edema. (**b1**) T2-weighted (3500/18) coronal MR image shows a fan-shaped bright signal intensity of edema (*arrow*). (**b2**) Gamma correction MR image shows the complete suppression of the edema signal intensity

small localized edema may present not harming trabeculae. Gamma correction suppressed small localized edema in the right femoral intercondylar fossa region due to motor vehicle accident in a 16-year-old male student (circle). The focal change was neatly suppressed in both coronal T1-weighted (460/26) MR image and ^{99m}Tc-HDP pinhole bone scan not showing any residual trabecular changes at all. We observed quite a similar phenomenon to manifest in large bone marrow edema as shown and proven by corroboratory T2 WT FS MR image (Fig. 15.7).

For information, the region of interest was initially characterized by base stain under lower power microscopy which showed characteristic H&E stain and the microfractures within the callused microfracture could be confirmed using high power scrutiny (Fig. 15.8). Trabecular microfracture was not demonstrated in every case. Indeed, some cases showed sharply defined thready fracture and others showed reminiscently, and still others showed none at all but with plain basophilic stain.

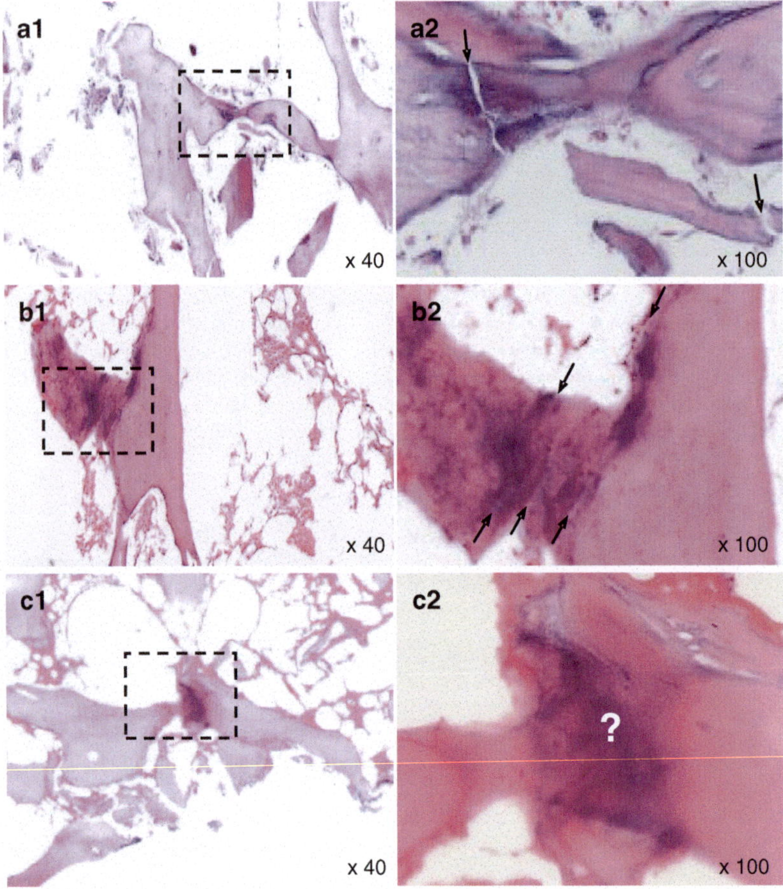

Fig. 15.8 Shapes and H&E stainability of trabecular microfractures may vary according to fracture type and stain quality. (**a1**) Low power view shows purple stain (*frame*). (**a2**) High power view shows distinctly defined lying down T-shape fracture with base stain. (**b1**) Scarcely defined fractures (*frame*). (**b2**) Moderately defined linear fractures with base stain. (**c1**) Only base stain without fracture. (**c2**) Even high power view failed to show fracture

References

Bahk YW, Chung YA. Gamma correction ^{99m}Tc-HDP scan diagnosis of trabecular microfracture and contusion. In: Bahk YW, editor. Combined scinitigraphic and radiographic diagnosis of bone and joint diseases including gamma correction interpretation. 5th ed. Berlin: Springer-Verlag; 2017. p. 649–88.

Bahk YW, Chung Y-A, Lee U-Y, et al. Gamma correction 99mTc-hydroxymethylene diphosphonate pinhole bone scan diagnosis and histopathological verification of trabecular contusion in young rats. Nucl Med Commun. 2016;37:988–91.

Bahk YW, Hwang SH, Lee UY, et al. Morphobiochemical diagnosis of acute trabecular microfractures using gamma correction Tc-99m HDP pinhole bone scan with histopathological verification. Medicine. 2017;96(45):e8419.

Eustace S, Keogh C, Blake M, et al. MR imaging of bone oedema: mechanisms and interpretation. Clin Radiol. 2001;56:4–12.

Francis MD, Ferguson DL, Tofe AJ, et al. Comparative evaluation of three diphosphonates: in vitro adsorption (C-14 labeled) and in vivo osteogenic uptake (Tc-99m complexed). J Nucl Med. 1980;21:1185–9.

Korompilias AV, Karantanas AH, Lykissas MG, et al. Bone marrow edema syndrome. Skelet Radiol. 2009;38:425–36.

Majkowski RS, Bannister GC, Miles AW. The effect of bleeding on the cement-bone interface. An experimental study. Clin Orthop Relat Res. 1994:293–7.

Mink JH, Deutch AL. Occult cartilage and bone injuries of the knee: detection, classification, and assessment with MR imaging. Radiology. 1989;170:823–9.

Pivonka P, Dunstan CR. Role of mathematical modeling in bone fracture healing. Bonekey Rep. 2012;1:221.

Rangger C, Kathrein A, Freund MC, et al. Bone bruise of the knee: histology and cryosections in 5 cases. Acta Orthop Scand. 1998;69:291–4.

Rosenson RS, McCormick A, Uretz EF. Distribution of blood viscosity values and biochemical correlates in healthy adults. Clin Chem. 1996;42:1189–95.

Salcianu IA, Bratu AM, Bondari S, et al. Bone marrow edema - premonitory sign in malignant hemopathies or nonspecific change? Romanian J Morphol Embryol. 2014;55:1079–84.

Thiryayi WA, Thiryayi SA, Freemont AJ. Histopathological perspective on bone marrow oedema, reactive bone change and haemorrhage. Eur J Radiol. 2008;67:62–7.

Yamamura M. Structural changes in jaw bone marrow after hemorrhagic infiltration. Kokubyo Gakkai Zasshi. 1994;61:207–20.

Zanetti M, Bruder E, Romero J, et al. Bone marrow edema pattern in osteoarthritic knees: correlation between MR imaging and histologic findings. Radiology. 2000;215:835–49.

16 Miscellanea of Gamma Correction Medical Imaging

Bone marrow edema (BME), bone marrow hemorrhage (BMH) and trabecular microfracture (TMF) are the essential triad of alive marrow bone changes, which homeostatically occur in trauma, sports injuries, osteoporosis, inflammation, infection, neoplasm, and even in daily physical activities and works (Salcianu et al. 2014). Such a phenomenon betokens that bone is insensitively yet vitally engaged with ceaseless active metabolic change to support and maintain thinking, respiration, and blood circulation in humans. Hence, the analytical differential assessment of each constituent of the triad is considered to be essential for the precise diagnosis of bone trabecular diseases at micrographic level. Fortunately, now CTMF (callused trabecular microfracture) can be clearly imaged by suppressing the blurry penumbra in BME and BMH using ACDSee-10 GCPBS (gamma correction pinhole bone scan) so that the triad can be precisely quantified (Fig. 16.1). Imaging wise, however, edema and hemorrhage are currently not distinguished from each other because both are equally suppressed by gamma correction. In order to overcome the difficulty, we adopted the mathematic categorization of ^{99m}Tc-HDP uptake values of BME and BMH using the NIH ImageJ densitometry in terms of "Arbitrary Unit (AU)" and found that there exists a significant difference between the AU values of edema and hemorrhage (Fig. 16.2). Practically, we could conveniently classify the AU of normal trabeculae to be ≤50 and AU of edema, hemorrhage, and trabecular microfracture to be 51–100, 101–150 AU, and ≥151, respectively (Bahk et al. 2019). Importantly, this classification is based on measurements of lesion size on naïve pinhole bone scan before gamma correction. Lately, a correlative analysis of the findings of seriated naïve pinhole bone scan (naive PBS) and GCPBS revealed that the diagnostic level of TMF in relation to BME and BMH is high.

Improved in young rat experiment (Bahk et al. 2016) as well as in patients (Bahk et al. 2017). It has also become evident that the NIH ImageJ densitometry (http://rsb.info.nih.gov/ij) is useful for the differential quantitation of ^{99m}Tc-HDP uptake in BME, BMH, and TMF. Additionally, the pixel measurement was found to be useful for the precise size assay of TMF. This combined technique of naïve-PBS-and-GCPBS assay, NIH ImageJ densitometry, and pixel measurement is termed visuospatial-mathematic assay (VSMA) (Bahk et al. 2019).

Now this section describes the results of VSMA for the differential diagnosis of BME, BMF, and TMF and histological validation. In addition, this discusses the usefulness and rationale of VSMA which enabled us to attain high-quality BME, BMH, and TMF images enabling precise anatomical and quantitative differential diagnosis possible as shown in (Fig. 16.2). For such differential diagnostic analysis 95 1-cm^2 areas of normal trabeculae (n = 16), BME

Y.-W. Bahk, *Imaging of Trabecular Microfracture and Bone Marrow Edema and Hemorrhage*,
https://doi.org/10.1007/978-981-15-4466-8_16

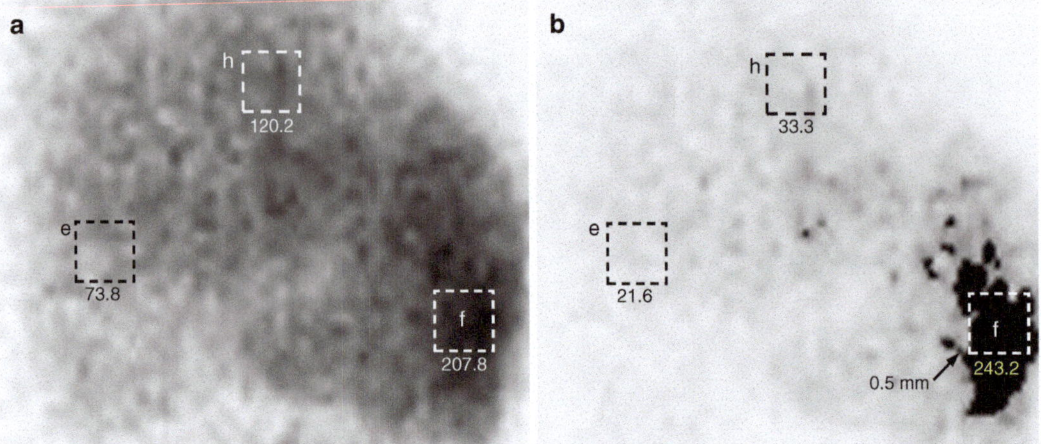

Fig. 16.1 Edema and hemorrhage can be differentiated using GCPBS and ImageJ densitometry. This is an adjusted view of Fig. 16.3 to present characteristically suppressed ^{99m}Tc-HDP uptake feature of edema and hemorrhage and highlighted uptake in fractures. (**a**) Naïve pinhole scan shows three 1-cm^2 areas of blurry tracer uptake of edema (*e*) and hemorrhage (*h*) and fracture (*f*) with AU values: the uptake in edema is 73.8, in hemorrhage is 120.2, and in fracture is 207.8. (**b**) Gamma correction suppresses edema and hemorrhage uptake highlighting fractures (*f*) with increased value of AU. Smallest fracture measures 500 μm in size. A large ovoid fracture is marked with f. Increased AU value in fracture after comma correction is due to enhanced signal-to-noise ratio

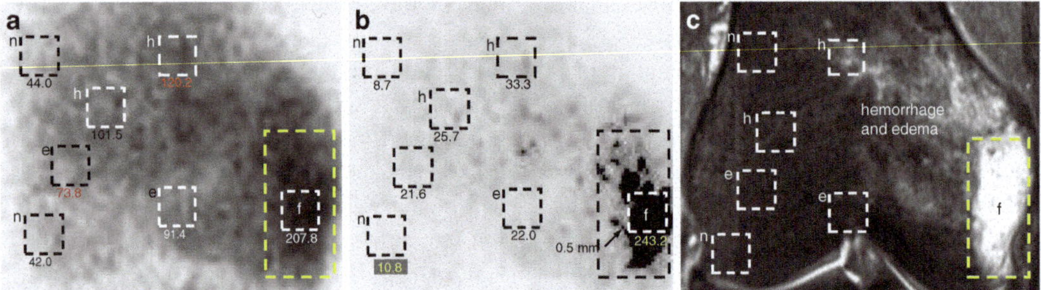

Fig. 16.2 Drifting edema and hemorrhage in cometary fracture involving left lateral femoral condyle in 71-year-old male. (**a**) Naïve PBS shows blurry mild and moderate tracer uptake in edema (*e*) and hemorrhage (*h*) (*1-cm^2 frame*) and intense tracer uptake in fracture (*yellow frame*). There are two areas each of edema, hemorrhage, and normal, and one fracture. Uptake value is 50 or less in normal site, 51–100 in edema, 101–150 in hemorrhage, and 151 or more in fracture. (**b**) Gamma correction suppresses uptake in edema, hemorrhage, and normal trabeculae and enhances uptake in fracture. Smallest fracture is 0.5 mm in size and lowermost AU value is 10.8 in normal trabeculae and highest AU is 243.2 in fracture. (**c**) Corroborative coronal FS T2 weighted MR image shows a large ovoid fracture with bright signal intensity (*yellow frame*) and two 1-cm^2 unit areas each of edema and hemorrhage with less bright signal intensities (*white frames*). It is to be remarked that ^{99m}Tc-HDP uptake value is significantly raised in fracture from 207.8 to 243.2 due to enhanced signal-to-noise ratio

($n = 44$), BMH ($n = 23$), and TMF ($n = 12$) were randomly sampled from seriated naïve PBS and GCPBS of 10 consecutive patients. Six cases were male and four were female with the age ranging from 16 to 71 years (average = 28.9 years). Cases covered the bones of the shoulder girdle ($n = 2$), hip ($n = 1$), knee ($n = 6$), and distal femoral shaft and condyles ($n = 1$) (Fig. 16.3). This study was approved by the Institutional Review Board to use only bone scan images without physical participation wavering consent. However, for the use of the surgical specimen of Fig. 16.1 patient agreed and signed an informed consent for its use.

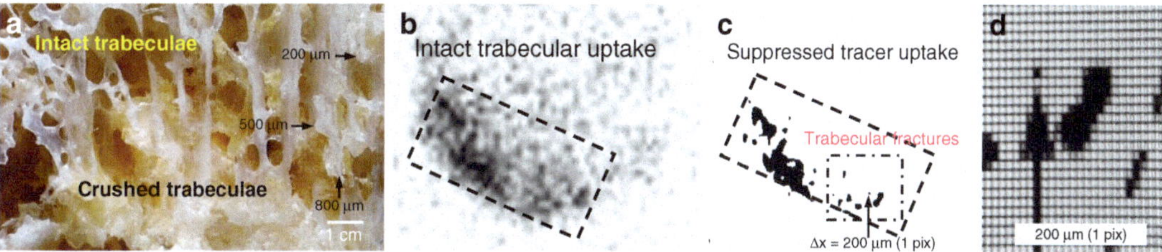

Fig. 16.3 ImageJ densitometry intensity value of ^{99m}Tc-HDP uptake in histopathologically verified intact trabeculae in surgically removed femoral head for bipolar prosthesis in a 72-year-old female patient. (**a**) Surgical micrograph shows trabecular microfractures with the smallest one measuring 200 **µ**m in size. There is crushed trabecular at the bottom. (**b**) Naïve ^{99m}Tc-HDP pinhole scan shows nonspecific blurry tracer uptake (frame). (**c**) ACDSee-10 gamma correction view demonstrates multiple microfractures with the smallest one measuring 200 **µ**m in size and two archipelagic fractures. (**d**) The pixel counting measurement using a 10× magnifying lens shows a single unit pixel involvement which measures 200 um

16.1 Diagnosis of Bone Marrow Edema and Hemorrhage and Trabecular Microfracture Using Naïve and Gamma Correction Pinhole Bone Scans, NIH ImageJ Densitometry, and Pixelized Microfracture Measurement

Bone marrow edema (BME), bone marrow hemorrhage (BMH), and trabecular microfracture (TMF) are the well-known triad of the fundamental marrow bone pathologies. Medical i\Imaging-wise, however, they are yet not differentially demonstrated and diagnosed because of methodological difficulty. In order to overcome this hurdle we prospectively designed and performed this seriated naïve and gamma correction pinhole bone scan (naïve PBS and GCPBS) study reinforced with the NIH ImageJ densitometry and pixelized microfracture measurement to individually make a specific diagnosis of BME, BMH, and TMF. Results were substantiated using the foregoing gold standard of gamma correction ^{99m}Tc-HDP pinhole bone scan finding and histopathology.

VSMA was performed in four technical steps: (1) BME, BMH, TMF, and normal trabeculae were differentially imaged using seriated naïve PBS and GCPBS; (2) the intensity of ^{99m}Tc-HDP uptake was measured using the NIH ImageJ densitometry in TMF in terms of Arbitrary Unit (AU); (3) the ^{99m}Tc-HDP uptake in TMF was measured using pixelized method; finally. (4) the fracture with unsuppressed bright signal intensity and two 1-cm^2 unit areas each of edema and hemorrhage with less bright signal intensities were assessed on corroborative coronal FS T2 weighted MR image. Actual techniques: (1) BME, BMH, TMF, and normal trabeculae were individually identified on seriated naïve PBS and GCPBS and naïve T2-weighted FS coronal MR image; (2) ^{99m}Tc-HDP uptake values were calculated using the ImageJ densitometry in terms of AU in each case; and finally (3) calculated values were categorized as 50 AU or less for normal trabeculae, 51–100 AU for BME, 101–150 AU for BMH, and 151 AU or more for microfracture. For result assessment the GraphPad prism software (San Diago, USA) statistics was performed confirming that the difference between normal and BME is significant ($P < 0.001$) and among BME, BMH, and TMF is highly significant ($P < 0.0001$; Fig. 16.4).

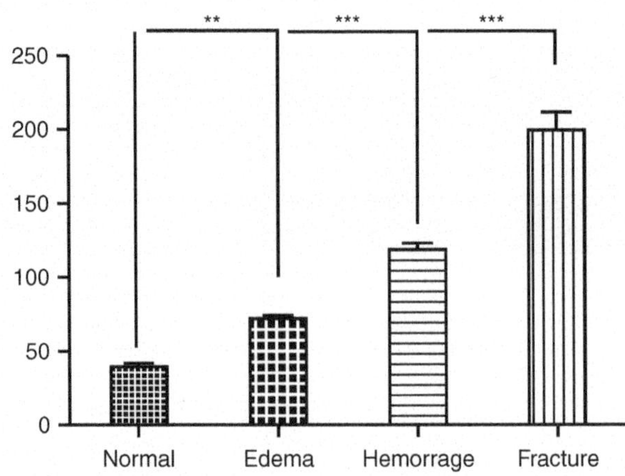

Fig. 16.4 Ninety five (95) sampled data were statistically treated using GraphPad Prism (San Diago, USA). Results were highly significant (** *P*-value was less than 0.001 and *** *P*-value was less than 0.000.1), respectively

16.2 Technique of Serial Naïve and Gamma Correction ^{99m}Tc-HDP Pinhole Bone Scan and Reference Conventional Radiography and Corroborative Coronal FS T2 Weighted MRI

Naïve PBS was taken using a conventional pinhole scan system (Siemens E-cam signature, Knoxville, Ohio, USA), which was equipped with a 4-mm pinhole collimator. The pinhole scan factors were 925–1110 MBq (25–30 mCi) ^{99m}Tc-HDP, 7-min scan time, and 12-cm pinhole-aperture-to-object distance to sufficiently encompass the bones of major joints including the shoulder, hip, knee, and distal tibiofibular syndesmosis. Gamma correction was performed by clicking the toolbars in the following sequence: Exposure and autoexposure to maximize uptake intensity and done and save with a new name. Then, exposure and image-brightness control were done by raising gamma values up to 95 starting from 50 (default value) and done and save the finished image with another name. The use of original naïve digital information and communications in medicine (DICOM) scan without image modification was strictly required. A reference conventional radiograph was taken in each case for fine topographic information of studied bones using a radiographic machine (Siemens Axiom Aristo MX, Erlangen, Germany). Exposure factors were 65–70 kVp and 35–40 mAs at 1-m source–image distance. Additionally, naïve corroborative coronal FS T2 weighted MR image (e.g., 3.500/18 for knee) was taken using 1.5-T Magnetom Avanto, Siemens, Erlangen, Germany (Figs. 16.2 and 16.3).

16.3 ImageJ Densitometry of ^{99m}Tc-HDP Uptake Measurement in Bone Marrow Edema and Hemorrhage and Trabecular Microfracture on Serial Naive and Gamma Correction Pinhole Bone Scans

The NIH ImageJ densitometry was performed in each case to categorically quantify ^{99m}Tc-HDP uptake value in BME, BMH, and TMF as presented in seriated naïve and gamma correction pinhole bone scans. Actually, ^{99m}Tc-HDP uptake intensity was calculated using the ImageJ densitometry in the randomly sampled 95 1-cm^2 areas of normal trabeculae (n = 16), BME (n = 44), BMH (n = 23), and TMF (n = 12). We found that the Arbitrary Unit (AU) of ImageJ densitometry itself was suited to differentially assess ^{99m}Tc-HDP uptake values in BME, BMH, and TMF (Bahk et al. 2019).

16.4 Mathematic Calculation of Callused Trabecular Microfracture with Unsuppressed ^{99m}Tc-HDP Uptake

The size of the individual TMF with unsuppressed ^{99m}Tc-HDP uptake was calculated using pixelized method [NIH.[4] Each micro-spot was appointed as a region of interest. The image profile is presented in a line spread function denoting the signal intensity of the applied line. The y-axis of image profile is signal intensity and the x-axis profile shows pixel number. In order to efficiently measure the full width at half maximum (FWHM), matrix size was expanded to 512 × 512. Because of the increased number of pixels, the signal intensity value was assigned by interpolation at the expanded bin, which does not have a signal intensity value. In order to interpolate the between bins, the Gaussian curve fitting method was checked using the in-house MATLAB code (Jung et al. 2016). The equation of the Gaussian curve fitting was as below:

$$y(x) = \frac{1}{\sigma\sqrt{2\pi}} \exp\left[-\frac{(x-x_0)^2}{2\sigma^2}\right]$$

y = interpolated value
x = original frame value
x_0 = mean value of the frame value
σ = standard deviation

16.5 Measurement of Different ^{99m}Tc-HDP Uptake of Bone Marrow Edema and Hemorrhage Using NIH ImageJ Densitometry and Histopathological Validation and Statistical Analysis

Imaging wise, the distinction of BME from BMH is an unfinished hard task, which needs many endeavor. Gamma correction is useless since it suppresses the tracer uptake equally in both BME and BMH. However, the recent attentive use of the ImageJ densitometry of tracer uptake intensity of NIH (Bahk et al. 2019) shed light on the precise quantitation of the differential ^{99m}Tc-HDP uptake intensities in acute BME and BMH as well as callused trabecular fractures. Differential NIH ImageJ uptake values can now distinguish edema from hemorrhage when 1-cm^2 region of interest is calculated in terms of AU on seriated naïve PBS and GCPBS (Fig. 16.3). For histopathological validation, we first performed rat study using traumatized bone marrow (Fig. 16.5) (Bahk et al. 2016) and it was successively followed by the study of operatively removed specimens of the femoral neck fracture in patients (Fig. 16.6) (Bahk et al. 2017). On the other hand, in an attempt to imaging-wise differentiate edema, hemorrhage, and CTMF the difference of the values of NIH ImageJ densitometry in terms of Arbitrary Unit (AU) (http://rsb.info.nih.gov/ij) was assessed to find that there exists a statistically significant difference among edema, hemorrhage, and CTMF (Bahk et al. 2019). ^{99m}Tc-HDP uptake intensity was individually measured in each case using the NIH ImageJ densitometry method in randomly sampled 95 1-cm^2 areas of abnormal and normal trabeculae in 10 consecutive naïve PBS. The attained value was designated as Arbitrary Unit (AU). Ninety five 1-cm^2 areas included BME (n = 44), BMH (n = 23), TMF (n = 12), and normal trabeculae (n = 16). Measurements were effectually performed in all except one outlier in TMF. The AU value of this TMF on naïve PBS was 142.4 but it recovered to 155.6 after gamma correction. As mentioned above the marrow space hemorrhage dips CTMF and additively injures already broken or contused trabeculae. The injuriousness of the hemorrhage with viscous blood, phagocytic neutrophils and monocyte, and the other blood ingredients is considered to be not negligible. Actually, the viscosity of edema is 1.27 ± 0.06 mPa.s, whereas that of hemorrhagic blood is 3.26 ± 0.43 mPa.s (Rosenson et al. 1996).

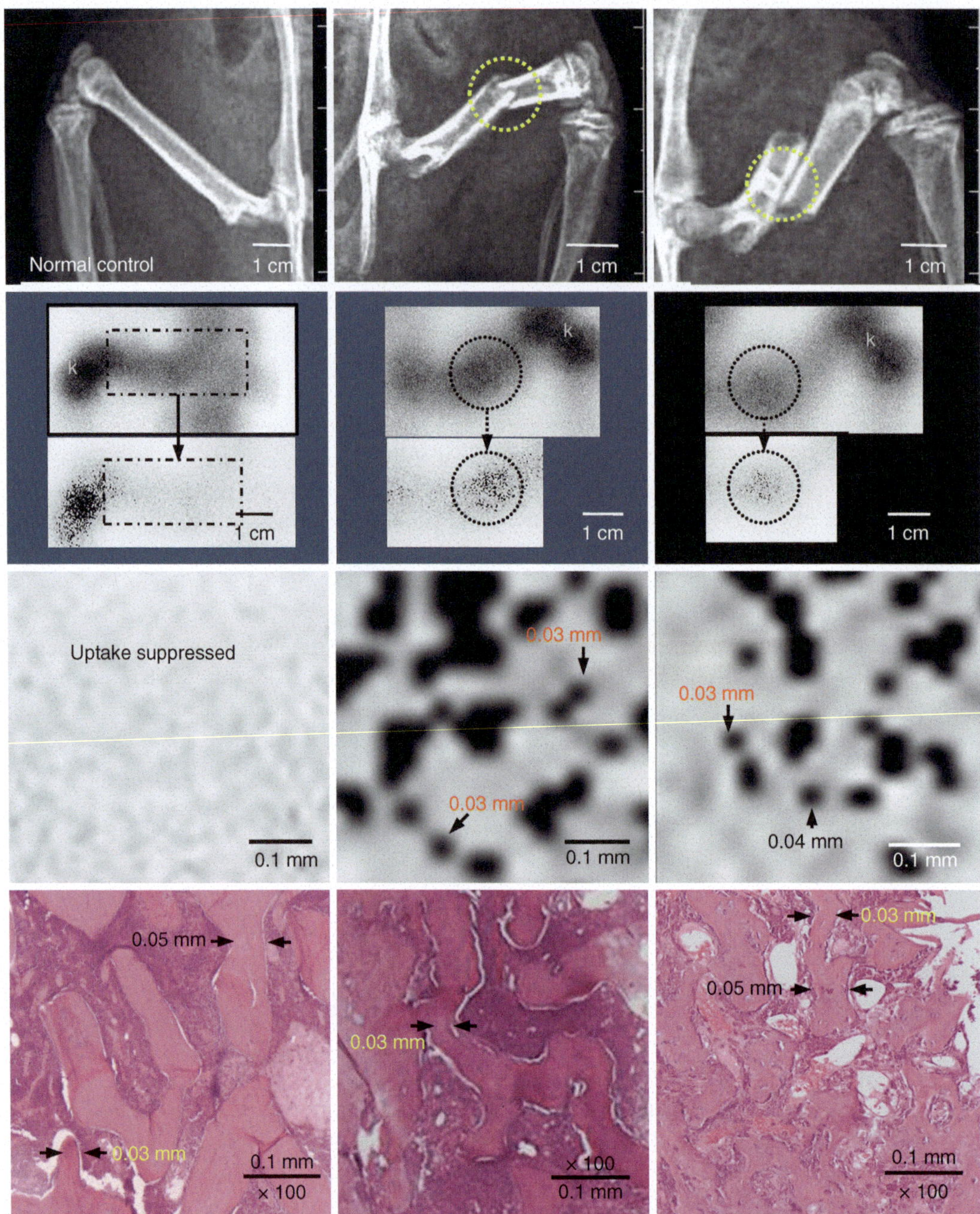

Fig. 16.5 Top panel: Radiographs of a normal control rat and two rats with femoral shaft fracture induced by a freely falling iron ball. Second panel: Upper image is naïve pinhole scan and lower image is ACDSee-7 gamma correction pinhole scan. Gamma correction view shows trabecular injuries. Third panel: ×50 magnified gamma correction views show suppressed ^{99m}Tc-HDP uptake in normal rat and callused trabecular microfractures with the smallest one measuring 30 **μ**m in size. Bottom panel: H&E stain shows normal trabeculae in control rat and endosteal rimming with hemorrhage in injured rats

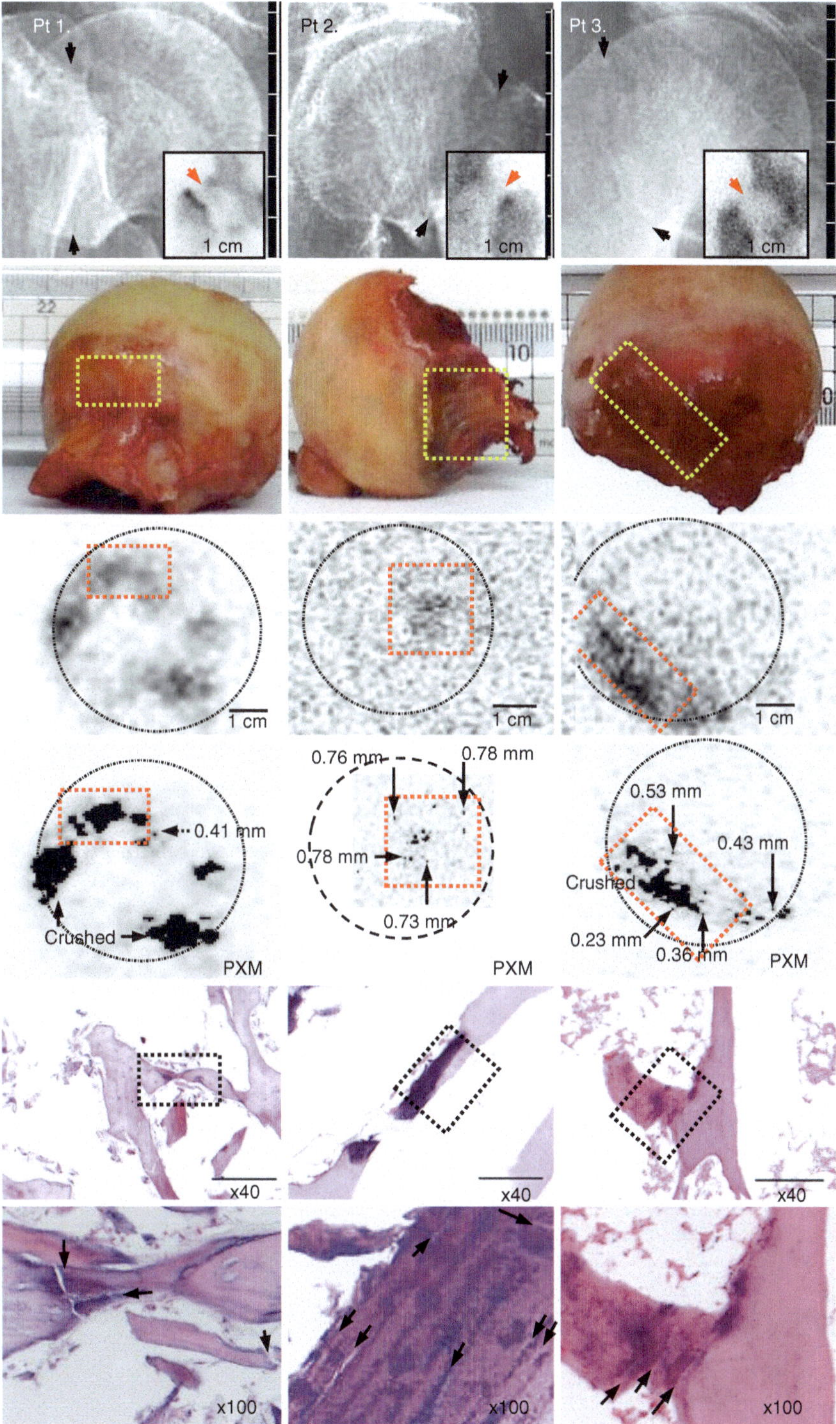

Fig. 16.6 Patients, examinations, and results. Top panel: Preoperative AP radiographs show femoral neck fracture (*arrow*). Inset is ^{99m}Tc-HDP pinhole bone scan showing avascular photopenia (*red arrow*). Second panel: Fresh surgically removed femoral heads show femoral neck fracture with a ruler for basic size measurement and the selection of ROI (*frame*). Third panel: Naive pinhole scans of specimen show nonspecific blurry tracer uptake (*red frame*). Fourth panel: Post GCPBS show unwashed high tracer uptake in pinpoint, speckled, rod-like, geographic, and crushed fractures. Size was measured using pixelized method (PXM). Note that the tracer uptake in normal and edema and/or hemorrhage is suppressed. Fifth panel: 40× H&E stain shows trabecular microfractures with callus formation. Bottom panel: 100× H&E stain shows linear microfractures

16.6 Differentiation of Bone Marrow Edema from Bone Marrow Hemorrhage Using NIH ImageJ Densitometry

Imaging-wise, bone marrow edema (BME) was hardly differentiated from bone marrow hemorrhage (BMH) although they may more often than not side by side co-occur in bone diseases. We attempted to differentiate BME from BMH first by unaided visual observation of naïve pinhole scan and ImageJ densitometric AU (http://rsb.info.nih.gov.ij; Bahk et al. 2019) assessment of tracer uptake values of edema and hemorrhage as measured in 1-cm^2 area on gamma correction pinhole scan (Fig. 16.3). ^{99m}Tc-HDP uptake intensity value was individually measured in terms of AU in 1-cm^2 area. Figure 16.2 was the utmost simplified version of Fig. 16.3 to emphatically highlight the visually observed difference of BME and BMH with differential AU values. Actually, the edema was presented as 1-cm^2 area of low tracer uptake on naïve PBS and the hemorrhage was presented as 1-cm^2 area of moderate tracer uptake. The mathematically calculated AU values were, for example, 73.8 in edema, 120.2 AU in hemorrhage, and 207.8 in fracture. Typically, GCPBS presented the fracture uptake remarkably raised to 243.2 (Fig. 16.3b). Corroborative fat suppression proton density MR image (3500/18) showed a similar difference in terms of signal intensity (Fig. 16.3c). Here, it is remarked that AU value will become to be significantly increased in a fracture on the post-gamma correction view because of raised signal-to-noise ratio, e.g., from 207.8 to 243.2.

16.7 Edema Is Suppressed by Gamma Correction and Innocuous to Intact Bone Trabeculae Regardless of Extent

The pure edema demonstrated by ^{99m}Tc-MDP pinhole bone scan can be neatly suppressed by gamma correction regardless of extent as proven by gamma correction T1 weighted MRI or T2 weighted mode. The smallest size of edema we came across was 2 cm in area (Fig. 16.6) and the largest was 5.5 × 6.5 cm (Fig. 16.7). Edema did not injure trabeculae inciting only mild ^{99m}Tc-HDP uptake that was cleanly suppressed by gamma correction, especially the ACDSee-10 version. The smallest edema happened to occur in the intercondylar fossa region and the largest one in the femoral condyle. Edemas were incited by a motor vehicle accident in both cases. The smallest one occurred in a 16-year-old male student and the largest one in a 24-year-old male. ImageJ uptake intensity was 56.8 AU which was in the lowermost value range for edema in the first case. The uptake intensity of the larger case was heterogeneous but all were equally suppressed cleanly.

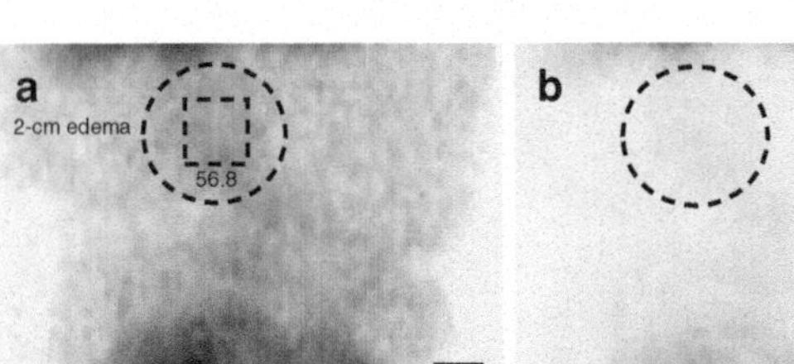

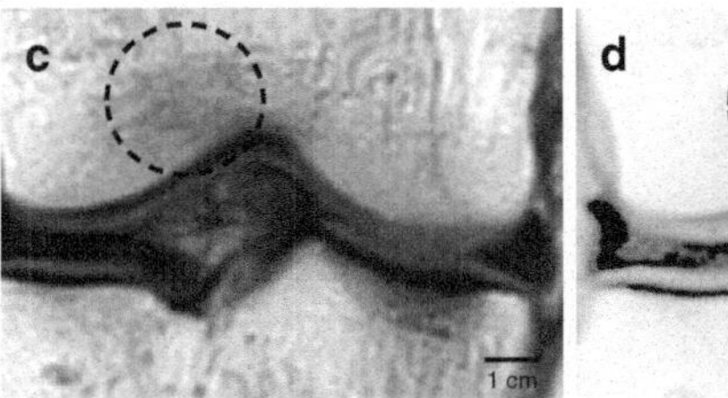

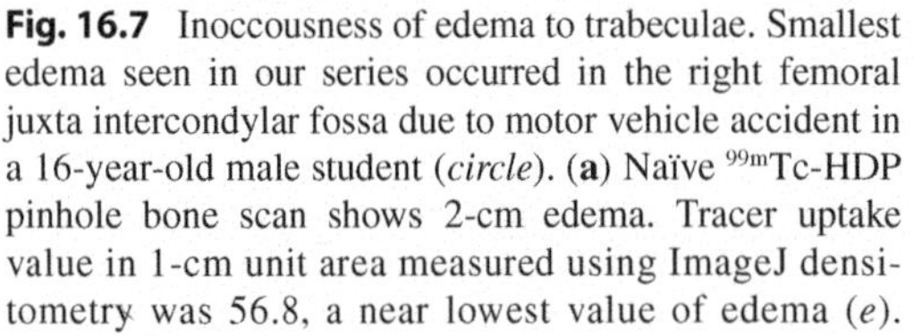

Fig. 16.7 Inoccousness of edema to trabeculae. Smallest edema seen in our series occurred in the right femoral juxta intercondylar fossa due to motor vehicle accident in a 16-year-old male student (*circle*). (**a**) Naïve ^{99m}Tc-HDP pinhole bone scan shows 2-cm edema. Tracer uptake value in 1-cm unit area measured using ImageJ densitometry was 56.8, a near lowest value of edema (*e*). (**b**) Gamma correction view shows suppression out of tracer uptake (*circle*). (**c**) Corroborative coronal T1-weighted (460/26) MR image shows edema with dark signal intensity (*circle*). (**d**) Gamma correction MR image shows suppression of dark signal MR intensity of edema with no architectural change (*circle*)

16.8 Discriminative NIH ImageJ Densitometry Values of ^{99m}Tc-HDP Uptake in Bone Marrow Edema and Hemorrhage and Callused Trabecular Microfracture

We investigated the discriminative value of ^{99m}Tc-HDP uptake calculated using the NIH ImageJ densitometry in seriated naïve PBS and GCPBS of 10 consecutive adult patients (Bahk et al. 2019). Conveniently, the uptake values calculated by this method could be classified into four categories; 50 AU or less for normal trabeculae, from 51 to100 AU for BME, from 101 to150 AU for BMH, and 151 AU or more for TMF. Our adoption of such an AU system of ImageJ densitometry to BME, BMH, and TMF was found useful as a quantitative scalar of ^{99m}Tc-HDP uptake. As shown in Fig. 16.3 the four different tracer uptake patterns were recognized; they were normal, edematous, hemorrhagic, and microfractured with thereto properly designated AU.

16.9 H&E Stain Validation of Additive Bone Marrow Hemorrhage which Injures Already Fractured Trabeculae with Unsuppressed Enhanced Tracer Uptake

Hemorrhage is considered to bathe and additively injure already fractured trabeculae by the phagocytic actions of neutrophils and monocyte and other irritating blood ingredients. TMF heals by osteoneogenesis that takes place in the form of callus and/or endosteal rimming onto which ^{99m}Tc-HDP was actively incorporated (Fig. 16.9).

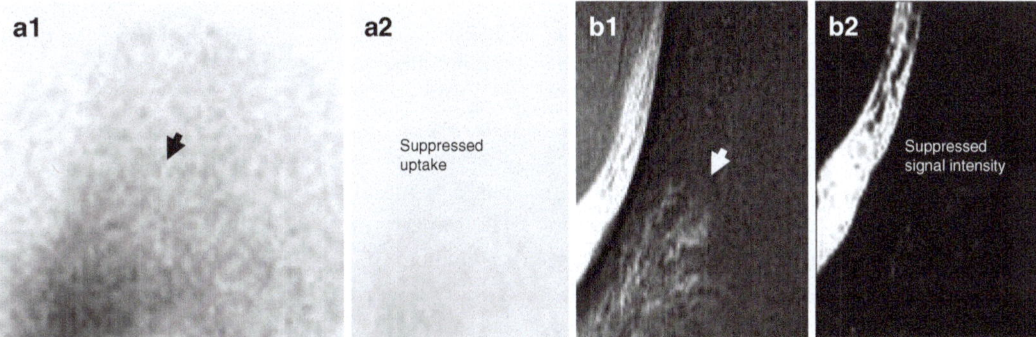

Fig. 16.8 Suppression of a large fan-shaped bone marrow edema in the left medial femoral condyle incited by motor vehicle contusion in a 24-year-old male. (**a1**) Naïve ^{99m}Tc-HDP pinhole scan shows large heterogeneous edema with increased tracer uptake (*arrow*). (**a2**) Gamma correction view shows the complete suppression of edema. (**b1**) T2-weighted (3500/18) coronal MR image shows a fan-shaped bright signal intensity of edema (*arrow*). (**b2**) Gamma correction MR image also shows complete suppression of the edema signal intensity

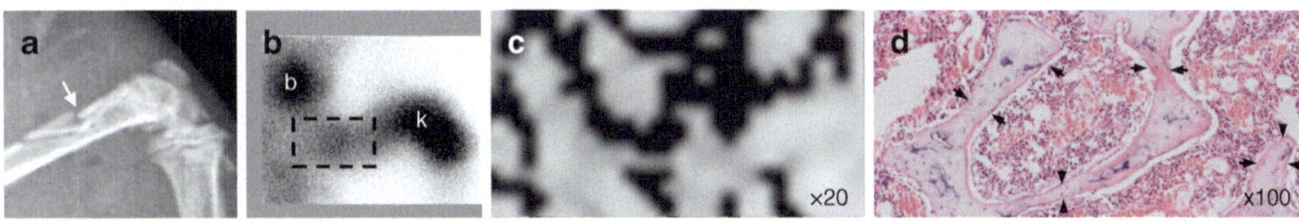

Fig. 16.9 Gamma correction distinguishes fracture from edema and hemorrhage in young rat. (**a**) Radiograph shows fracture (*arrow*). (**b**) Naive pinhole scan shows injured area (*frame*). *b* is bladder and *k* is knee. (**c**) ACDSee-7 gamma correction view shows enhanced tracer uptake in endosteal rimming. (**d**) H&E stain confirms endosteal rimming with hemorrhage

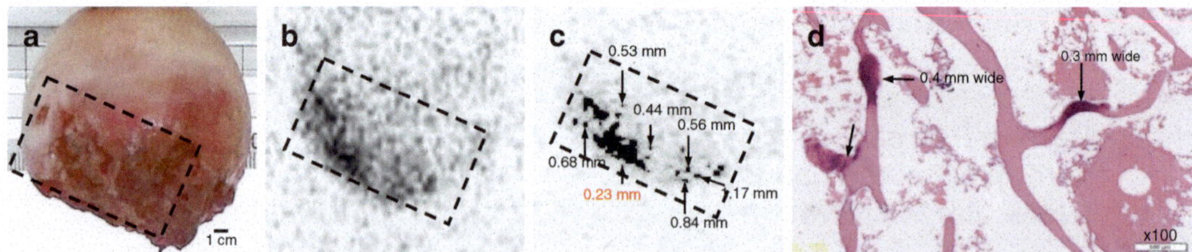

Fig. 16.10 Histological verification of unsuppressed tracer uptake in trabecular microfractures in femoral head. Femoral head was removed for prosthesis. (**a**) Surgical specimen shows a roughened fracture surface with seed-pearly microfractures (*frame*). (**b**) Naïve ^{99m}Tc-HDP pinhole scan shows nonspecific blurry tracer uptake (*frame*). (**c**) Gamma correction view shows suppressed blurry tracer uptake highlighting microfractures. Sizes were measured using pixelized method. The smallest microfracture measured 0.23 mm in size. (**d**) H&E stain shows a base stained microfractures (*arrows*)

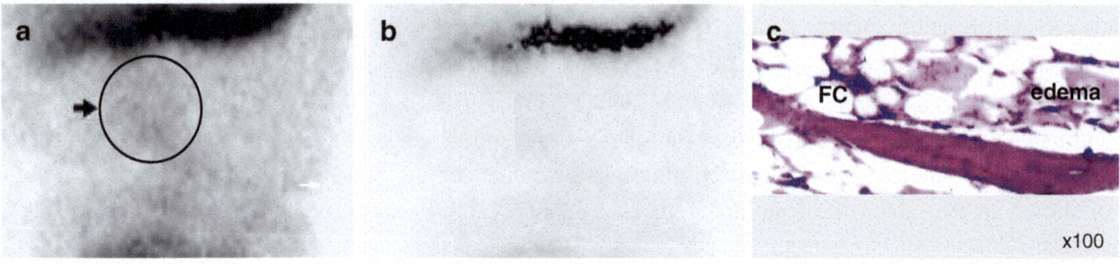

Fig. 16.11 Inoccuousness of simple edema to trabeculae due to motor vehicle accident in a 16-year-old male student (*circle*). (**a**) Naïve pinhole scan of right femoral condylar fossa shows faint edema uptake (*arrow*). (**b**) Gamma correction completely suppresses edema. (**c**) H&E stain shows edema and fat cells with intact trabeculae (from teaching file). FC is a fat cell

Endosteal rimming can be demonstrated with high unsuppressed tracer uptake in reactive trabeculae which are long club-shaped when longitudinally imaged, short club-shaped when obliquely imaged, and nodular when transaxially imaged. On the other hand, TMF is imaged as pinpoint, speckled, bar-like, linear, and archipelagic high ^{99m}Tc-HDP uptake, which were not suppressed by gamma correction (Fig. 16.10). All those trabecular changes were histologically verified.

16.10 Innocuousness of Edema to Trabeculae

Mere BME does not injure intact trabeculae (Fig. 16.11), but BMH is associated with or accompanied by trabecular microfracture or endosteal rimming with unsuppressed high ^{99m}Tc-HDP uptake in rat (Fig. 16.9; Bahk et al. 2016) and patient (Fig. 16.10; Bahk et al. 2017). Such a difference is interpreted to denote that simple edema is innocuous not injuring intact trabeculae (Fig. 16.11).

References

Bahk YW, Chung YA, Lee UY, et al. Gamma correction ^{99m}Tc-hydroxymethylene diphosphonate pinhole bone scan diagnosis and histopathological verification of trabecular contusion in young rats. Nucl Med Commun. 2016;37:988–91.

Bahk YW, Hwang SH, Lee UY, et al. Morphobiochemical diagnosis of acute trabecular microfractures using gamma correction Tc-99m HDP pinhole bone scan with histopathological verification. Medicine. 2017;96:e8419. https://doi.org/10.1097/MD.0000000000008419.

Bahk YW, Kim EE, Chung YA, et al. Precise differential diagnosis of acute bone marrow edema and hemorrhage and trabecular microfractures using naïve and gamma correction pinhole bone scans. J Int Med Res. 2019;47(4):1493–503. https://doi.org/10.1177/0300060518819910.

Jung J-Y, Cheon GJ, Lee Y-S, et al. Pixelized measurement of ^{99m}Tc-HDP micro particles formed in gamma correction phantom pinhole scan: a reference study. Nucl Med Mol Imaging. 2016; 50:207–12.

Rosenson RS, McCormick A, Uretz EF. Distribution of blood viscosity values and biochemical correlates in healthy adults. Clin Chem. 1996;42:1189–95.

Salcianu IA, Bratu AM, Bondari S, et al. Bone marrow edema–premonitory sign in malignant hemopathies or nonspecific change? Romanian J Morphol Embryol. 2014;55:1079–84.

Index

Y.-W. Bahk, *Imaging of Trabecular Microfracture and Bone Marrow Edema and Hemorrhage*,
https://doi.org/10.1007/978-981-15-4466-8

The manufacturer's authorised representative in the EU is Springer Nature Customer Service Centre GmbH, Europaplatz 3, 69115 Heidelberg, Germany. If you have any concerns regarding our products, please contact ProductSafety@springernature.com

Printed and bound by CPI Group (UK) Ltd, Croydon, CR0 4YY
15/07/2026
02167649-0004